Examining the State of the Science of Mammalian Embryo Model Systems

PROCEEDINGS OF A WORKSHOP

Siobhan Addie, Meredith Hackmann, Anna Nicholson,
and Sarah H. Beachy, *Rapporteurs*

Board on Health Sciences Policy

Health and Medicine Division

The National Academies of
SCIENCES · ENGINEERING · MEDICINE

THE NATIONAL ACADEMIES PRESS
Washington, DC
www.nap.edu

THE NATIONAL ACADEMIES PRESS 500 Fifth Street, NW Washington, DC 20001

This activity was supported by a contract between the National Academy of Sciences and the National Institutes of Health (Contract No. HHSN263201800029I; Order No. 75N98019F00854, P00001). Any opinions, findings, conclusions, or recommendations expressed in this publication do not necessarily reflect the views of any organization or agency that provided support for the project.

International Standard Book Number-13: 978-0-309-67668-7
International Standard Book Number-10: 0-309-67668-1
Digital Object Identifier: https://doi.org/10.17226/25779

Additional copies of this publication are available from the National Academies Press, 500 Fifth Street, NW, Keck 360, Washington, DC 20001; (800) 624-6242 or (202) 334-3313; http://www.nap.edu.

Printed in the United States of America

Suggested citation: National Academies of Sciences, Engineering, and Medicine. 2020. *Examining the state of the science of mammalian embryo model systems: Proceedings of a workshop*. Washington, DC: The National Academies Press. https://doi.org/10.17226/25779.

The National Academies of
SCIENCES • ENGINEERING • MEDICINE

Consensus Study Reports published by the National Academies of Sciences, Engineering, and Medicine document the evidence-based consensus on the study's statement of task by an authoring committee of experts. Reports typically include findings, conclusions, and recommendations based on information gathered by the committee and the committee's deliberations. Each report has been subjected to a rigorous and independent peer-review process, and it represents the position of the National Academies on the statement of task.

Proceedings published by the National Academies of Sciences, Engineering, and Medicine chronicle the presentations and discussions at a workshop, symposium, or other event convened by the National Academies. The statements and opinions contained in proceedings are those of the participants and are not endorsed by other participants, the planning committee, or the National Academies.

For information about other products and activities of the National Academies, please visit www.nationalacademies.org/about/whatwedo.

PLANNING COMMITTEE FOR A WORKSHOP ON EXAMINING THE STATE OF THE SCIENCE OF MAMMALIAN EMBRYO MODEL SYSTEMS[1]

MARTIN PERA (*Co-Chair*), Professor, The Jackson Laboratory
JANET ROSSANT (*Co-Chair*), Senior Scientist, Developmental and Stem Cell Biology, The Hospital for Sick Children
RICHARD BEHRINGER, Professor, Department of Genetics, Division of Basic Science Research, The University of Texas MD Anderson Cancer Center
AMANDER CLARK, Professor and Chair, Department of Molecular, Cell and Developmental Biology, University of California, Los Angeles
ARNOLD KRIEGSTEIN, John Bowes Distinguished Professor in Stem Cell and Tissue Biology and Founding Director, Eli & Edythe Broad Center of Regeneration Medicine and Stem Cell Research, University of California, San Francisco
MANA PARAST, Professor in Residence, Pathology, University of California, San Diego
RENEE REIJO PERA, Vice President of Research and Economic Development, California Polytechnic State University

Board on Health Sciences Policy Staff

SARAH H. BEACHY, Senior Program Officer
SIOBHAN ADDIE, Program Officer
MEREDITH HACKMANN, Associate Program Officer
MICHAEL BERRIOS, Research Associate
KELLY CHOI, Senior Program Assistant
BRIDGET BOREL, Program Coordinator
ANDREW M. POPE, Senior Board Director

[1]The National Academies of Sciences, Engineering, and Medicine's planning committees are solely responsible for organizing the workshop, identifying topics, and choosing speakers. The responsibility for the published proceedings of a workshop rests with the workshop rapporteurs and the institution.

Reviewers

This Proceedings of a Workshop was reviewed in draft form by individuals chosen for their diverse perspectives and technical expertise. The purpose of this independent review is to provide candid and critical comments that will assist the National Academies of Sciences, Engineering, and Medicine in making each published proceedings as sound as possible and to ensure that it meets the institutional standards for quality, objectivity, evidence, and responsiveness to the charge. The review comments and draft manuscript remain confidential to protect the integrity of the process.

We thank the following individuals for their review of this proceedings:

ANA M. FERARAS, The National Academies of Sciences, Engineering, and Medicine
JACK MOSHER, International Society for Stem Cell Research
LILIANNA SOLNICA-KREZEL, Washington University in St. Louis

Although the reviewers listed above provided many constructive comments and suggestions, they were not asked to endorse the content of the proceedings nor did they see the final draft before its release. The review of this proceedings was overseen by **LESLIE BENET,** University of California, San Francisco. He was responsible for making certain that an independent examination of this proceedings was carried out in accordance with standards of the National Academies and that all review comments were carefully considered. Responsibility for the final content rests entirely with the rapporteurs and the National Academies.

Contents

Boxes and Figures

BOXES

FIGURES

Acronyms and Abbreviations

BLIMP1	B-lymphocyte-induced maturation protein 1
BMP4	bone morphogenetic protein 4
BRA	BRACHYURY
CAG	cytosine-adenine-guanine
CDX2	caudal type homeobox 2
CG	chorionic gonadotropin
CGA	alpha peptide of chorionic gonadotropin
CGB	beta peptide of chorionic gonadotropin
CTB	cytotrophoblast
DHEA-S	dehydroepiandrosterone sulfate
EB	embryoid body
EGF	epidermal growth factor
EpiSC	epiblast-derived stem cell
EPSC	extended- or expanded-potential pluripotent stem cell
ESC	embryonic stem cell
EVT	extravillous trophoblast
FGF	fibroblast growth factor
GATA3	GATA binding protein 3
GCM1	glial cells missing transcription factor 1
GDF	growth differentiation factor

hCG	human chorionic gonadotropin
hESC	human embryonic stem cell
HFEA	Human Fertilization and Embryology Authority
HLA-G	human leukocyte antigen-G
hPSC	human pluripotent stem cell
ICM	inner cell mass
IGF1	insulin growth factor
iPSC	induced pluripotent stem cell
IVF	in vitro fertilization
IWP2	Inhibitor of Wnt Production-2
KLF4	Krüppel-like factor 4
MEK/ERK	mitogen-activated protein kinase/extracellular-signal-regulated kinase
MMP	matrix metalloproteinase
nEND	naïve extraembryonic endoderm (cells)
NIH	National Institutes of Health
Nodal	Nodal Growth Differentiation Factor
OCT4	octamer-binding transcription factor 4
PE	primitive endoderm
PGT-A	pre-implantation genetic testing for aneuploidy
PI3K	phosphoinositide 3-kinase
PSC	pluripotent stem cell
REC	Research Ethics Committee
SNAIL	Zinc finger protein SNAI1
SNP	single-nucleotide polymorphism
SOX	SRY-related HMG-box family of genes
STB	syncytiotrophoblast
TDGF1	teratocarcinoma-derived growth factor 1
TE	trophectoderm
TGFβ	transforming growth factor beta
TSC	trophoblast stem cell
VGLL1	vestigial like family member 1

XEN	extraembryonic endoderm
YAP1	yes-associated protein 1
ysTE	yolk sac trophectoderm

1

Introduction and Overview

Early human embryo development is studied for a variety of reasons, including to better understand our fundamental origins, with the goal of using that information to provide insights into infertility, implantation, and placental development and to apply that knowledge to improve assisted reproductive technologies such as in vitro fertilization (IVF). The use of embryo models to study human embryogenesis can contribute new knowledge about an essential stage of human development that is otherwise inaccessible (see the section on the Current State of Regulation of Research on Human Embryo Models in Hyun et al., 2020). These embryo models can provide important information to guide infertility treatments, prevent disease, and create organs that could be used for pharmacologic screening or possibly even for transplantation.

A host of technical breakthroughs in modeling early embryonic development has been achieved in the past few years. A new technique of geometrical confinement has enabled the self-organization of human stem cells to be modeled in two dimensions (2D) using micropatterns (Warmflash et al., 2014). Three-dimensional (3D) culturing systems use hydrogels that modify the physical environment of embryonic development, allowing for the use of mouse stem cells to create 3D models of features of the embryo prior to implantation to illuminate the process of placental formation and elucidate the reasons for the high rates of early human embryo loss and human placental anomalies (Rivron et al., 2018b). Human pluripotent stem cells grown in microfluidic systems offer opportunities to study early post-implantation biology with even greater control and reproducibility than 3D modeling (Zheng et al., 2019). CRISPR-Cas9 techniques have revolutionized gene editing in human cells and can be used to study the genetics underlying early developmental defects. Similarly, the advent of single-cell omics has been pivotal in understanding the genetic features of early embryos, while developmental genetics has generated a wealth of new information about developmentally important genes.

OVERVIEW OF THE WORKSHOP

Because of the recent advances in embryo modeling techniques, and at the request of the Office of Science Policy in the Office of the Director at the National Institutes of Health (NIH), the National Academies of Sciences, Engineering, and Medicine appointed a planning committee to develop and host a 1-day public workshop[1] that would explore the state of the science of mammalian embryo model systems. The workshop, which took place on January 17, 2020, featured a combination of presentations, panels, and general discussions, during which panelists and participants offered a broad range of perspectives. The workshop began with a survey of the developments that have laid the groundwork for the field, then focused on opportunities and challenges for future work with embryo model systems. Presentations and discussions covered topics such as the characteristics of advanced mammalian embryo model systems, the differences between various mammalian embryo model systems and bona fide mammalian embryos, and the differences between mammalian embryo model systems and mammalian "embryoid bodies," which arise via aggregation of stem cells but do not recapitulate regular organization. Participants considered whether embryo model systems—especially those that use nonhuman primate cells—can be used to predict the function of systems made with human cells. They also considered the functionality and organismal potential of the model systems—that is, whether embryo model systems have organismal potential if they lack trophoblast cells or other extraembryonic cell types. Presentations provided an overview of the current state of the science of in vitro development of human trophoblast cells. As requested by NIH, the discussions at the workshop focused on the state of the science, not on policy or ethical implications.

[1]This workshop was organized by an independent planning committee whose role was limited to identification of the topics and speakers. This Proceedings of a Workshop was prepared by the rapporteurs as a factual summary of the presentations and discussion that took place at the workshop. Statements, recommendations, and opinions expressed are those of individual presenters and participants and are not endorsed or verified by the National Academies of Sciences, Engineering, and Medicine, and they should not be construed as reflecting any group consensus. The workshop agenda, speaker biographies, planning committee Statement of Task, and a list of attendees can be found in Appendixes A, B, C, and D, respectively.

OPPORTUNITIES AND CHALLENGES WITH STEM CELL–BASED EMBRYO MODELS

Janet Rossant, a senior scientist in the Program in Developmental and Stem Cell Biology at The Hospital for Sick Children, University of Toronto, delivered an opening keynote that focused on the unique aspects of human embryology and opportunities and challenges with stem cell–based embryo models. Opportunities already exist to generate partial or more complete stem cell–derived human embryo models. However, she said, embarking on this human model pathway will require careful consideration of the similarities and differences between mouse and human systems in order to select the appropriate cell type for developing human models. Furthermore, it will require aligning directly with events in the human embryo itself, either via culture in vitro or in comparison with nonhuman primate models.

Comparison of Human and Mouse Development

Rossant explained why mouse models are not sufficient for understanding early human development. Although human and mouse development have many similarities, the processes are morphologically and molecularly distinct (Rossant and Tam, 2017). To illustrate, she compared the timelines of human and mouse development. In both species the blastocyst is the first major differentiated state of the embryo, containing three cell types—trophectoderm, epiblast, and hypoblast. Many of the genes that are involved in specifying the three cell types in the mouse are also involved in the human blastocyst. However, there are differences in the time of activation of the genes that specify cell fate, which likely relates to a difference in the timing of zygote genome activation. Lineage-specific gene expression cannot begin until zygotic genome activation has occurred, which happens at a later developmental timepoint in the human than the mouse. Much larger morphological differences between the two species occur post-implantation. Regenerative medicine will be one of the areas that will benefit from a better understanding of the similarities and differences between human and mouse embryos and their derived stem cells, she added.

Timing of Blastocyst Lineage Commitment in Mouse and Human

The timing of blastocyst lineage commitment is different in mouse and human development, Rossant said. Studies of the timing of the commitment of inner cell mass (ICM) in trophectoderm in the blastocyst have established that mouse lineage commitment occurs in trophectoderm before the ICM, although both cell lineages are committed by the blastocyst stage (Posfai et al., 2017; Wigger et al., 2017). That is, if the cells are taken apart and reaggregated, they cannot regenerate a blastocyst. She described some of the relevant gene expression and signaling pathways involved in this process. In addition to early cell biases, the Hippo/YAP and fibroblast growth factor (FGF) signaling pathways are critical to final cell fate specification in the mouse blastocyst. Less information is available on blastocyst lineage commitment in humans, although some studies suggest that human early blastocyst cells remain uncommitted to lineage (De Paepe et al., 2013).

Timing of Gene Expression

The timing of the expression of key transcription factors differs between mouse and human, Rossant said, and those factors may also differ in function between the species. For instance, single-cell RNA sequencing shows that many key genes in the mouse early embryo are conserved in humans, but there are also divergent lineage-specific genes (Blakeley et al., 2015; Petropoulos et al., 2016). For example, caudal type homeobox 2 (CDX2), which is presumed to be important for trophectoderm, does not begin expression in the human until after blastocyst formation, which gives rise to questions about how it can drive cell fate specification (Niakan and Eggan, 2013). Furthermore, knock-out gene editing studies suggest that OCT4 may play a much different role in human development than in the mouse (Fogarty et al., 2017). It has been established that the morphogenesis of the human blastocyst precedes lineage specification, but it is still unknown whether CDX2 is important to trophectoderm or whether Hippo signaling is required. Rossant explained that these differences are important because they may relate to the derivation of different types of pluripotent stem cells from the blastocyst.

Differences in Post-Implantation Morphogenesis

Additional morphological distinctions emerge post-implantation in human and mouse development, Rossant said. The major difference between the mouse and the human post-implantation is the formation of the extra-embryonic ectoderm from the polar trophectoderm, which proliferates and pushes the ICM into the blastocoel to form a cup-shaped epiblast. The polar trophectoderm does not proliferate in this way in humans; instead of a cup shape, the epiblast is shaped like a flat sheet. In vitro outgrowths of human embryos across the implantation period (i.e., less than 14 days) have demonstrated morphogenesis of the post-implantation embryos (Deglincerti et al., 2016; Shahbazi et al., 2016), although the human embryos were still largely disorganized. Two laboratories have recently developed techniques to extend in vitro cultures of cynomolgus monkey embryos for longer than

14 days in the hope of achieving better morphology, she added (Ma et al., 2019; Niu et al., 2019).

Replacing Human Embryos with Self-Organizing Stem Cell Cultures

The use of human or nonhuman primate embryos as model systems will not be sufficient, Rossant said. The use of human embryos can be considered ethically challenging in many regions, while nonhuman primate embryos are expensive and only available in limited research centers. These challenges have led researchers to replace human embryos with self-organizing stem cell model systems in order to study development without the use of embryos. The use of self-organizing embryo stem cell cultures began and is most advanced with the mouse system, she explained. Fortunately, the mouse system has three lineage-specific stem cell lines that represent the three lineages of the blastocyst: trophectoderm, epiblast, and primitive endoderm. This provides a starting population of cells that can be combined to model some of the events of blastocyst formation and early post-implantation development. Embryonic stem cells (ESCs) come from the ICM of the blastocyst, Rossant said, and express the pluripotency genes. When placed back in the chimera, they contribute to the fetus but usually not to the placenta or the yolk sac. Trophoblast stem cells (TSCs) arise from the trophectoderm and have a different growth factor requirement which enables them to grow indefinitely in culture; they make placental tissues later in development. Extraembryonic endoderm (XEN) cells can also grow indefinitely in culture and contribute only to yolk sac endoderm. One laboratory has already been able to take these three cell types from the blastocyst and recombine them to form 3D "artificial" mouse embryo models which look like early post-implantation embryos, and to model early interactions between these cell lineages which are critical in later development (Sozen et al., 2018). Nicolas Rivron's laboratory has been able to create mini blastoids that resemble the mouse blastocyst by combining ESCs and TSCs and allowing them to reaggregate such that TSCs form an outer trophectoderm layer (Rivron et al., 2018b). These efforts demonstrate that the use of stem cells in mouse systems has the potential to mimic pre-implantation and early post-implantation development by aggregate systems, she explained.

Use of Mouse Stem Cells for Model Generation

Rossant provided updates on progress in the use of mouse stem cells for model generation, with the caveat that the three original ES, TS, and XEN cell types are not necessarily completely equivalent to the three cell types of the blastocyst and that more work is needed to mimic the three lineages of the mouse blastocyst. Nicolas Rivron's laboratory has shown that TSCs that express higher levels of CDX2 are more like the polar trophectoderm (TE) and are thus more likely to accurately represent the cells that would reconstitute a blastoid rather than post-implantation trophoblast (Aldeguer et al., 2019). Josh Brickman's laboratory has demonstrated that culture conditions from ESCs can make naïve extraembryonic endoderm (nEND) cells that are closer to the primitive endoderm than XEN cells, suggesting that they may provide a better system for embryo models (Anderson et al., 2017). Several laboratories have derived extended-potential stem cells that are purported to be able to generate extraembryonic tissues themselves; because they have an extended potential beyond pluripotent cells, they can generate epiblast and primitive endoderm when combined with TSCs to make a blastoid (Sozen et al., 2019). Extended-potential stem cells may also have the potential to make trophoblast-like cells as well, meaning that the extended-potential cells could make blastoids (Li et al., 2019).

Potential to Use Human Stem Cells for Embryo Models

To offer more context on the shift from mouse to human stem cells for embryo models,[2] Rossant provided a brief overview of the literature to date about what can be modeled with stem cells (Hyun et al., 2020). Mouse systems have been used for several years to model blastocyst formation and post-implantation interactions between the trophoblast, endoderm, and epiblast; ESCs have also been used to create gastrula-like structures. On the human side, there have been no reports of blastoid formation published to date, although studies have used micropattern cultures to model some of the events of gastrulation in 2D and 3D. Microfluidic systems have also been used to create small amniotic sac structures. Only ESCs have been used thus far in human models, Rossant said. She discussed whether naïve ES, TS, and XEN-type cells are available for use in human stem cell models.

Similarities Between Mouse and Human Stem Cells

Human naïve ESCs do exist and are the closest cell type to the epiblast or the blastocyst; thus, they may be good candidates for use in an embryo model, Rossant said. It has been suggested that the naïve state of ESCs in the human may be different than in the mouse. However, like mouse naïve ESCs, human naïve ESCs can grow in 2i LIF+FGFR inhibitor (Anderson et al., 2017). Human TSCs cannot be derived from blastocysts in humans

[2]Rossant noted that related ethical and regulatory issues were beyond the scope of the workshop, but a review is available in Hyun et al. (2020).

using mouse conditions, which involves activating FGF signaling. Because the early trophoblast in the human does not proliferate, it does not respond to FGF signaling in the embryo itself. However, good-quality TSCs have been generated from human blastocyst and early villus structures that express and have many of the properties of early placental cells (Okae et al., 2018). The lack of dependence on FGF in human TSCs indicates that a different set of signaling pathways is important in humans. The question remains as to whether there is a blastocyst-type TE cell to be found in humans or whether they do not exist, in which case human TSCs may be the best tools to monitor the state of development, Rossant said. It is possible to overexpress SOX7 (a member of the SRY-related HMG-box family of genes) (Seguin et al., 2008) as well as expressing other genes that would drive human ESCs toward primitive endoderm. Brickman's laboratory has been able to culture human nEND cells using the same conditions to make mouse nEND cells, which are posited to mimic the primitive endoderm and can be cultured indefinitely (Linneberg-Agerholm et al., 2019). The expanded-potential cells that have been reported in the mouse to produce trophoblast and primitive endoderm have also been reported in the human, using culture conditions similar to the mouse (Gao et al., 2019). Because these cells have similar properties to the mouse cells, there is great interest in whether they can produce blastoids as well.

Differences Between Mouse and Human Stem Cells

Rossant highlighted several differences between mouse and human stem cells. Although it appears that human naïve ESCs can be cultured in conditions similar to those used for mouse cells, the lineage status of the human cells is less clear. Naïve ESCs in the mouse are restricted to the epiblast lineage, so they do not normally make the other blastocyst cell types—many other factors need to be added to generate extended-potential cells. However, evidence suggests that human naïve ESCs may have some intrinsic extended potential; their expression profile shows similarity to some stages in early pre-implantation development, as well as to the epiblast (Stirparo et al., 2018). Transposon expression and other properties of these cells have also been reported to be similar to cleavage stages (Theunissen and Jaenisch, 2017). Rossant noted that in humans, even the blastocyst stage shows late plasticity, with no lineage commitment. She surmised that this may explain why these naïve cells seem to have an extended potential: they are behaving like blastocyst cells. Data also suggest that human expanded-potential stem cells (Gao et al., 2019)—and naïve cells (Dong et al., 2020)—may be more readily able to generate TSCs in the appropriate culture conditions than mouse expanded-potential stem cells.

NEW MODELS MAY OFFER A NEW FRONTIER OF DATA

There has been enormous progress in the past 5 years in using cell culture systems to model mammalian embryonic development, said Martin Pera, a professor at The Jackson Laboratory in Bar Harbor, Maine, and member of the workshop planning committee. Technologies to replicate cell specification and differentiation events have been available for much longer, but novel systems have opened up a new frontier in providing the opportunity to model cell patterning and morphogenetic events in space and time. With these advances comes the potential to better understand the earliest stages of human development, he said, and the advances may offer the means to explore and ultimately intervene to address disorders that may have their origin in early embryonic development. At the level of basic science, these systems can not only shed light on fundamental questions about our human origins, but elucidate similarities and differences in embryonic development across species. These systems can also contribute to a better understanding of the origin of germ cells in order to address issues of infertility.

New data are also emerging from studies characterizing the molecular attributes of embryos from the mouse, human, and nonhuman primate. Moving the field of mammalian embryology forward with these transformative new systems and techniques will involve venturing down new avenues of research to explore how embryo research interacts with stem cell models to harness the vast potential of pluripotent cells. It will also require conducting comparative cross-species studies of early embryonic development and investigating the nature of the broad range of cell types that can now be generated and manipulated, M. Pera said.

ORGANIZATION OF THE PROCEEDINGS OF A WORKSHOP

Following this introductory chapter, Chapter 2 explores the current state of mammalian embryo model systems, the use of pluripotent stem cells to generate those models, and the potential benefits and limitations of using these models for studying human embryonic development. Speakers discussed the molecular mechanisms of lineage specification in human embryos, described the development of embryo models, and considered the clinical implications of modeling pre-implantation embryo development. Chapter 3 examines the development of extraembryonic lineages and the impact of those lineages on human embryo model systems, featuring presentations on modeling trophoblast differentiation using pluripotent stem cells and molecular innovation in the human trophoblast lineage. Chapter 4 provides an overview of cutting-edge novel systems that have been developed to model human embryos from stem cells. Speakers described techniques for modeling attachment and self-organization in human embryonic development using 3D models and 2D micropatterns, systems for modeling the pre-implantation embryo in 3D, and the use of microfluidic systems to model the peri-implantation embryo. Chapter 5 summarizes the workshop session on comparative embryonic development across species. Speakers explored mechanisms underlying pre-implantation chromosomal instability, systems to differentiate trophoblast from primate pluripotent cells, models of early neural crest formation in humans, and models of pre-implantation development generated from pluripotent stem cells with expanded potential. Finally, Chapter 6 summarizes the workshop's final panel discussion and closing keynote, which focused on future opportunities and challenges of mammalian embryo model systems.

2

Mammalian Embryo Research and Pluripotent Stem Cells

Important Points Highlighted by Individual Speakers

- Transcriptome analysis can be used to understand early human development, refine methods for understanding gene function in human embryos, and optimize the culture conditions for human embryonic stem cells and induced pluripotent stem cells. (Niakan)
- Insulin growth factor promotes the proliferation of the pluripotent epiblast in embryonic stem cells and, together with Nodal Growth Differentiation Factor (Nodal)/Activin, supports the derivation and maintenance of embryonic stem cells and induced pluripotent stem cells. (Niakan)
- Human and mouse embryos have distinct expression dynamics; for example, fibroblast growth factor and Nodal signaling may function differently in mouse and human pre-implantation development. (Niakan)
- Studying the early stages of human development is beneficial because it can lead to improved rates of success with in vitro fertilization (IVF) and a better understanding of human embryonic stem cells, which have self-renewal capacity and regenerative potential. (Niakan)
- Studying early post-implantation human development informs our understanding of human origins and elucidates how human development differs from other species. (Zernicka-Goetz)

- Three-dimensional model systems can mimic the early stages of development and be used to explore the mechanisms of embryo self-organization. (Zernicka-Goetz)
- Compared with other animals, human reproduction is markedly inefficient, with high rates of developmental arrest, aneuploidy, and implantation failure. IVF protocols provide a unique opportunity to observe the earliest stages of development and can help inform the development of embryo model systems. (Cook-Andersen)
- Studies of gene expression patterns and cell–cell communication networks in human blastocysts indicate that defective primitive endoderm development in embryos with poor morphology may be a common cause of implantation failure in humans. (Cook-Andersen)
- Studying pre-implantation human embryo development is critical for identifying reproductive inefficiencies that are unique to humans and for applying this knowledge to advance clinical reproductive sciences. (Cook-Andersen)

The first session of the workshop focused on mammalian embryo research and pluripotent stem cells with the aim of exploring the characteristics of mammalian embryo model systems and the potential benefits and limitations to using these models for studying human embryonic development. The session was moderated by Renee Reijo Pera, the vice president of Research and Economic Development at California Polytechnic State University, and featured presentations on the molecular mechanisms of lineage specification in human embryos, human and synthetic models of human development after implantation, and the clinical implications of studying pre-implantation human development.

MOLECULAR MECHANISMS OF LINEAGE SPECIFICATION IN HUMAN EMBRYOS

Kathy Niakan, a group leader at the Francis Crick Institute, a biomedical research institute in London, spoke about molecular mechanisms of lineage specification in human embryos. Little is known about how the first cell types that emerge in a human embryo become specialized in fate and function, so her laboratory uses transcriptome analysis to understand early human development and to refine methods for understanding gene function in human embryos. Currently, this knowledge is used to rationally design and optimize culture conditions for human embryonic stem cells (hESCs) and induced pluripotent stem cells (iPSCs). The members of Niakan's lab hope to use the knowledge to identify biomarkers of successful embryo development with the aim of improving in vitro fertilization (IVF) culture conditions. In her presentation, Niakan highlighted distinct expression dynamics in human versus mouse embryos, explained why human pluripotent stem cell culture conditions need to be improved, and described how genome editing can contribute to the understanding of early human development. She also provided an overview of the regulatory framework for human embryonic research in the United Kingdom for the purposes of understanding the environment in which the work was conducted (see Box 2-1).

Rationale for Studying Human Pre-Implantation Development

Niakan's laboratory focuses on understanding the mechanisms of early lineage specification in humans during the first 7 days of development, which encompasses the time immediately after the egg is fertilized until it forms a ball of approximately 200 cells called the blastocyst. The human blastocyst is composed predominantly of placental progenitor cells collectively called the trophectoderm, Niakan said. The human blastocyst also contains endoderm cells, which are the precursors of the yolk sac. Only a small subset of cells in the developing human pre-implantation

BOX 2-1
Regulatory Framework for Human Embryonic Research in the United Kingdom

The United Kingdom has two distinct national regulatory authorities, the Human Fertilization and Embryology Authority (HFEA) and the Health Research Authority, which oversees National Research Ethics Committees (RECs). HFEA and RECs both have members with diverse backgrounds, including members of the public. Researchers apply for project approval from regional ethics committees, which operate at arm's length from their institutes, and also apply to the executive and license committee of HFEA. Within HFEA there are also separate advisory committees with specialized expertise: a Scientific and Clinical Advances Advisory Committee, a Horizon Scanning Panel, and an Ethics and Law Review Group. All research is subject to review every 3 years—including scientific peer review—as well as to annual audits and inspections.

SOURCE: Kathy Niakan workshop presentation, January 17, 2020.

blastocyst—about 5 percent—have the unique potential to give rise to the entire embryo proper or the fetus. These are called the epiblast progenitor cells, and they express a key transcription factor called octamer-binding transcription factor 4 (OCT4).

In addition to fundamentally informing our understanding of human biology, studying early lineage specification and human pre-implantation development also has clinical implications, Niakan said. Most human IVF embryos will fail to develop to form a blastocyst, fail to implant, or fail to develop beyond 3 months. Across all IVF clinics in the United Kingdom, the aggregated ongoing pregnancy rate, irrespective of age, is only about 11 percent (Koot et al., 2012). Studying these early stages of development may lead to a better understanding of the conditions that human embryos need to continue development and help identify more accurate predictors of success in embryos used for transfer in treatment. Studying these early stages of development is also important for stem cell biology, because hESCs can be established from epiblast progenitor cells in the blastocyst. These cells have tremendous regenerative potential, Niakan said, because they can self-renew and could theoretically be directed to differentiate into any cell type; hence, the importance of understanding how pluripotency is established and maintained.

Distinct Expression Dynamics in Human Versus Mouse Embryos

To better understand the mechanisms of lineage specification, Niakan's laboratory performed single-cell RNA sequencing to catalog which genes are expressed throughout the various pre-implantation stages of human development and then compared this list of genes with the corresponding one for the mouse, which remains the most important model organism for comparative analysis. A comparison of these transcriptome analyses for the two species revealed striking differences in the temporal gene expression patterns between the homologous or potentially orthologous genes in the two species (Blakeley et al., 2015). Differences in cell-type-specific expression were also found among other genes that may have more conserved expression patterns, including POU class 5 homeobox 1 (*POU5F1*)—which encodes the key transcription factor OCT4—as well as Krüppel-like factor 4 (*KLF4*). The expression of both of those genes is detectable much earlier within mouse development than within human development, she said.

Early Lineage Specification in Mice and Humans

In order to delve further into what is known about lineage specification in humans, Niakan first described what is known about how lineages are specified in mice. In the mouse, the first lineage decision occurs at the morula stage, when outer cells initiate a program that ultimately gives rise to trophectoderm cells and inner cells subsequently segregate to form the primitive endoderm or the pluripotent epiblast. The mechanisms that underlie this first lineage decision in the mouse are thought to be shaped by differences in polarization state that influence cell fate (Nishioka et al., 2009). An anterior polarity complex comprising atypical protein kinase C and PAR proteins[1] sequesters angiomotin to the cell membrane. This prevents the activation of Hippo kinases and allows the yes-associated protein 1 (YAP1) transcription factor to translocate into the nucleus, where it accumulates and activates trophectoderm genes. This process does not occur in the inner cells; instead, the Hippo kinases phosphorylate YAP and prevent it from translocating into the nucleus to drive trophectoderm cell initiation. Niakan's laboratory is currently investigating whether these components are also expressed in human pre-implantation embryos.

Niakan explained that research on the first lineage segregation event serves to benchmark what is likely the next segregation event (i.e., segregation of the pluripotent epiblast from the primitive endoderm). In the mouse model it is well established that the pluripotent epiblast secretes a ligand fibroblast growth factor (FGF) that binds to an FGF receptor enriched on primitive endoderm-fated cells. Blocking either that receptor or the downstream mitogen-activated protein kinase/extracellular-signal-regulated kinase (MEK/ERK) pathway prevents the initiation of genes associated with primitive endoderm differentiation (Yamanaka et al., 2010). This finding has been used to improve mouse embryonic stem cell culture conditions in the naïve pluripotent stem cell state (Ying et al., 2008). For reasons not yet understood, hESCs seem to require FGF for their self-renewal (Thomson et al., 1998).

Rationale for Improving Human Pluripotent Stem Cell Culture

Decades of research using hESCs have been transformative for our understanding of human biology, Niakan said. However, there are important justifications for continued research into how pluripotent epiblast cells form and how to refine hESC culture conditions using actual human embryos, she continued. Decades of work with iPSCs and ESCs have been valuable, but pluripotent stem cell culture conditions need to be improved to more closely approximate the processes of normal embryonic development. Some pluripotent stem cells—especially human naïve cells—that are established in cultures have epigenetic abnormalities, such as abnormalities in genomic

[1]PAR proteins are a highly conserved group of proteins across the metazoan that control cell polarity during development.

imprinting, which may preclude their use in understanding certain aspects of human biology. Improving these culture methods might also decrease known line-to-line variabilities between human ESCs and iPSCs as well as facilitating the generation of mature cell types with greater phenotypic fidelity to in vivo counterparts. On a pragmatic level, improving human pluripotent stem cell culture conditions may also be more cost permissive, especially for large-scale experiments such as three-dimensional (3D) cell-suspension cultures, she added.

Nodal Signaling and Insulin Growth Factor in Pre-Implantation Development

Niakan's laboratory returned to its transcriptome datasets to investigate signaling pathways that could be modulated to rationally design human pluripotent culture conditions that more closely recapitulate the niche. They identified that a number of components of the Nodal Growth Differentiation Factor (Nodal) signaling pathway are transcribed specifically in the embryonic epiblast, including Nodal and the co-factors growth differentiation factor 3 (GDF3) and teratocarcinoma-derived growth factor 1 (TDGF1, which encodes Cripto). Next, they posited that blocking the Activin-receptor-like kinases involved in the Nodal signaling pathway would have a consequence for downstream NANOG[2] expression, which has been demonstrated to be affected in hESCs following inhibition of this pathway. Indeed, treating human embryos with inhibitors of Nodal signaling led to a loss of downstream NANOG expression; the same effect was not observed in mouse embryos treated with the same inhibitors, suggesting potential differences. Thus, it appears that Nodal signaling may be necessary for the maintenance of NANOG in human epithelial cells (Blakeley et al., 2015). The signaling pathway for insulin growth factor (IGF1)—active phosphoinositide 3-kinase (PI3K)/AKT/mTOR signaling—was also found to be active in human embryos (Wamaitha et al., 2020). By stimulating the Nodal signaling pathway with IGF1 in novel culture conditions, they were able to derive hESCs directly from embryos and reprogram fibroblasts into iPSCs. These cells express key pluripotency-associated transcription factors and cell-surface antigens and can be directed to differentiate into a variety of different lineages. Having established the novel culture conditions, Niakan and colleagues then assessed the transcriptional similarities and differences and used the novel culture conditions to make strides toward moving the cells closer to the embryonic epiblast. They found that irrespective of the culture conditions, established hESCs are somewhat transcrip-

[2]NANOG is a transcription factor that helps embryonic stem cells maintain pluripotency by suppressing cell determination factors.

tionally different from the pluripotent epiblast, despite some similarities to the embryonic epiblast (Wamaitha et al., 2020). Niakan added that even naïve hESCs are still somewhat transcriptionally different, even though they have upregulated many genes that are uniquely expressed in the embryonic epiblast. This suggests that further refinements of human pluripotent stem cell culture conditions are needed and that a basic understanding of how the embryonic epiblast develops in human embryos may provide key insights into how to make further improvements.

Based on this work, Niakan said she believes that FGF and Nodal signaling may differ in how they function in mouse and human preimplantation development. Her team found that IGF1 promotes proliferation of the pluripotent epiblast in ES cells and that Nodal (Activin) together with IGF1 supports the derivation and maintenance of hESCs and iPSCs. IGF1 likely functions as a proliferative factor and is not involved in lineage segregation, she added. It is not yet clear how the epiblast and the primitive endoderm diverge in humans, and this is likely a distinct mechanism compared to the mouse.

Use of Genome Editing to Understand Early Human Development

Genome editing approaches are another way to better understand early human development, Niakan said. Her laboratory has targeted OCT4 in human embryos using CRISPR-Cas9 genome editing as a proof-of-principle in order to determine if these methods are useful in understanding human biology (Fogarty et al., 2017). She said that they screened various methods in hESCs and in mouse embryos to optimize their techniques before they targeted human embryos. It appears that human embryos need OCT4 to correctly form a blastocyst (Fogarty et al., 2017). Human embryos in which OCT4 was targeted were significantly less likely to develop to the blastocyst stage—despite embryos initiating blastocyst formation, the blastocysts cannot be maintained. Genotyping and transcriptome analysis revealed that the OCT4-targeted cells are transcriptionally distinct from unedited cells with respect to NANOG expression. OCT4-targeted human embryos lacked detectable NANOG expression, while in mouse embryos, OCT4-null mutant mouse embryos retained NANOG expression, Niakan said. This suggests that NANOG is differentially regulated between the species. In addition to the retention of NANOG expression in OCT4-null mutant mouse embryos, the expression of placental markers (e.g., CDX2) is retained (Frum et al., 2013). In fact, OCT4-null mutant mouse embryos plated in mouse embryonic culture conditions preferentially gave rise to trophoblast or placental outgrowths. In contrast, trophectoderm development is compromised in OCT4-targeted human embryos (Fogarty et al., 2017). This suggests that OCT4 is a negative regulator of the placental program in the mouse and a positive regulator of the program in the human. Altogether, this suggests that while some developmental programs may be conserved across species, there may be important distinctions in early embryogenesis, underscoring the importance of studying human embryos directly, Niakan said.

BUILDING EMBRYO MODELS TO STUDY HUMAN DEVELOPMENT

Magdalena Zernicka-Goetz, a professor of mammalian development and stem cell biology at the University of Cambridge and the Bren Professor of Biology and Biological Engineering at the California Institute of Technology, described her laboratory's work on early post-implantation human embryo development that led to the development of synthetic 3D stem cell models. She cited two reasons for studying early human development: (1) because it is the initiation of human life and (2) because of basic interest in understanding how human development is different than other models, particularly in the mouse. Research into early human development also provides a new frontier of opportunity for understanding why only about 30 percent of human pregnancies are successful, she said. During the preclinical stage, an estimated 30 percent of human pregnancies fail prior to the implantation phase of development and another 30 percent of pregnancies fail around the time of implantation or soon after; yet another 10 percent of pregnancies are lost to miscarriage (Macklon et al., 2002). The embryos themselves—rather than the endometrium—are typically the cause of the pregnancy loss. Around 85 percent of recovered embryos have chromosomal abnormalities.

Early Post-Implantation Human Embryo Development: Research Aims

Zernicka-Goetz outlined four research aims that her laboratory has pursued in the realm of early post-implantation human embryo development. The first aim was to develop the conditions that would allow human embryos to be cultured in vitro beyond implantation, in order to understand the morphogenesis of the human embryo at the time of implantation and soon after. In addition to uncovering the sequence of morphogenetic steps that an embryo undergoes, another aim of developing this model system was to create a molecular map of transitions that occur in the human embryo during those early stages using single-cell transcriptomic analysis. A third aim was to study the development of aneuploid and mosaic human embryos by investigating the developmental consequences of specific aneuploidies during post-implantation development. Mosaic embryos were of particular interest because they contain both normal and abnormal cells, giving rise to questions about what happens to those abnormal cells when they are surrounded by normal cells in early development—for example, whether their development is normal and whether those cells can be manipulated by normal cells in ways that might lead to cell death, as Zernicka-Goetz's laboratory recently demonstrated in the mouse. Using the knowledge gained from achieving the first three research aims, the lab has developed four different 3D model systems to mimic the early stages of development and explore the mechanisms of embryo self-organization.

Modeling Human Embryo Development After Implantation

Zernicka-Goetz explained that until recently human post-implantation development could not be studied directly. Knowledge of this stage was limited to the analysis of a small number of embryos that had developed in vivo and were recovered after hysterectomy (Hertig et al., 1956). Her laboratory considered two alternative paths for exploring this phase of development: (1) to develop a system to culture human embryos beyond day 7 in vitro that is as similar as possible to human development in vivo and (2) to develop a system to model human development with stem cells. They had already developed a system to culture mouse blastocysts in vitro through the implantation stages into the post-implantation gastrulation stage, which initiates anterior-posterior polarity (Bedzhov and Zernicka-Goetz, 2014; Bedzhov et al., 2014; Morris et al., 2012), and they found that the same system could be used to culture human embryos from the blastocyst stage onwards (Deglincerti et al., 2016; Shahbazi et al., 2016). Today, many groups are using this stem cell–based system to identify the sequential morphogenic steps involved in early post-implantation human embryo development (Shahbazi and Zernicka-Goetz, 2018; Zhou et al., 2019). Zernicka-Goetz added that, in addition to morphogenesis, this stem cell culture system can also reveal mechanisms that underlie the sequential stages of post-implantation development and drive different tissues to develop the unique characteristics that enable future development of the fetus, placenta, and yolk sac.

Molecular Mapping of Human Embryos

Having the stem cell–based developmental system in place, Zernicka-Goetz's laboratory looked at the genes that are expressed at different stages in various tissues to understand the molecular fate of those tissues. Focusing first on day 9 and day 11, they isolated cells and identified epiblast, hypoblast, cytotrophoblast, and syncytiotrophoblast tissues based on markers of gene expression. Zernicka-Goetz described this study as important in providing the molecular fingerprint for morphogenic events observed in early embryonic development. Her lab will now be using this approach to understand signaling interactions between the tissues.

Developmental Consequences of Specific Aneuploidies

The culture conditions developed to study normal human embryo development can also be used to look at aneuploid embryos and identify the developmental consequences of specific aneuploidies, Zernicka-Goetz said. She maintained that this stem cell–based system has great potential to further our understanding of how genes on specific chromosomes contribute to the phenotype and behavior of trophectoderm, epiblast, and hypoblast. Using this method, she said, her lab will also be able to identify embryos that are misdiagnosed as aneuploid when they are actually mosaic.

Embryo Growth in the Stem Cell Culture System

Zernicka-Goetz explained how her lab determines whether the embryos are behaving normally in this model system. One method is to rely on established markers of in vivo developing embryos, but a clear indication that the embryos are behaving normally is that embryo growth is observed in the individual culture systems. In fact, embryo development is very simple prior to implantation—the embryo cleaves into smaller and smaller cells, albeit with a complex cell rate specification. Embryo growth does not begin until implantation, at which point all the tissues begin to proliferate, and major remodeling occurs. At days 7 and 8 the cells segregate into the epiblast and hypoblast lineages, marked by OCT4 and GATA6, respectively. At days 8 and 9 a group of epiblast cells forms the pre-amniotic cavity. Zernicka-Goetz and colleagues were able to mimic the formation of this cavity by culturing human stem cells in Matrigel, a 3D extracellular matrix (Bedzhov and Zernicka-Goetz, 2014; Shahbazi et al., 2017). They surrounded human ESCs with Matrigel, which allows the cells to become polarized. Upon polarization, the amniotic cavity is formed, she said. In this way, studying human stem cells elucidates the morphological transition for both the mouse and the human at this very early stage of development. Extraembryonic tissues begin to differentiate at days 10 and 11. Hypoblast tissue[3] forms the prospective yolk sac, and trophoblast tissue differentiates into cytotrophoblast and syncytiotrophoblast. Zernicka-Goetz described this study as a breakthrough in showing that human embryos can self-organize in vitro outside the body of the mother and said that this model system can be used to mimic natural human development in vitro, at least to a certain extent.

[3]Hypoblast tissue is the equivalent of primitive endoderm in the mouse.

Four 3D Stem Cell Models of Early Development

Zernicka-Goetz described how her laboratory has developed four 3D stem cell embryo model systems to generate embryo-like structures. To do so they applied the knowledge gleaned from observing the development of normal and abnormal embryos on morphological and molecular levels using their initial culture system. Their research aim was to inform the mechanistic understanding of development by reconstructing mammalian embryos using the building blocks of stem cells for three distinct tissues: ESCs from epiblast, extraembryonic endoderm (XEN) cells from primitive endoderm, and trophoblast stem cells (TSCs) from trophectoderm.

Pre-Implantation Blastocyst Model

In the first mouse model, Zernicka-Goetz and colleagues sought to mimic the formation of the pre-implantation blastocyst using expanded-potential ESCs, which can form both epiblast and primitive endoderm. TSCs were added to make a chimera of the two types of stem cells. The cells self-organized to form blastocyst-like structures (i.e., "blastoids") with all three constituent cell types (Li et al., 2019; Rivron et al., 2018b; Sozen et al., 2019). The advantage of this model is that it provides insight into the blastocyst stage, she said. The drawback is that the model does not develop very well to post-implantation stages, because it induces an implantation-like reaction but does not progress to post-implantation stages.

Peri-Implantation Blastocyst Model

The second 3D model developed by Zernicka-Goetz's laboratory was designed to look at the peri-implantation phase. Mouse or human ESCs are embedded in Matrigel and allowed to undergo polarization and lumenogenesis (Bedzhov and Zernicka-Goetz, 2014; Shahbaz et al., 2017). This model offers insights in the cellular and molecular mechanisms underlying mouse and human lumenogenesis, which opens up an amniotic cavity as well as the interrelationships between different pluripotent states and tissue architectures.

Post-Implantation Polarizing ETS Model[4]

Zernicka-Goetz noted that in normal embryonic development, ESCs are surrounded by extraembryonic cells to induce polarization. Their next

[4]The ETS model refers to an in vitro model that combines embryonic and extraembryonic stem cells on a 3D matrix. More details about the ETS model can be found in Harrison et al. (2017).

model was designed to mimic this phenomenon (Harrison et al., 2017). Mouse ESCs were combined with TSCs, leading to the formation of "ET embryos" composed of embryonic and extraembryonic compartments. These mouse ET embryos grow and appear similar to normal embryos. She remarked that this model provided important insights (e.g., that the processes of symmetry breaking, mesoderm specification, and primordial germ cell formation do not require the presence of the anterior signaling center that is normally involved in those processes).

Post-Implantation Embryo Model

The fourth model was designed to study the mechanisms that enable cells to communicate and self-assemble to create the embryo structure with all three compartments and therefore a model that can induce the formation of not only posterior but also anterior structures. To create this model system, Zernicka-Goetz's group combined mouse ESCs, TSCs, and XEN cells to build post-implantation-stage embryo models that look extremely similar to natural embryos (Sozen et al., 2018). This model makes it possible to study the principles directing self-organization leading up to initiation of gastrulation.

CLINICAL PERSPECTIVE ON PRE-IMPLANTATION HUMAN EMBRYO DEVELOPMENT

Heidi Cook-Andersen, an assistant professor of reproductive medicine at the University of California, San Diego, offered a clinical perspective on how studying pre-implantation human embryo development can elucidate inefficiencies in human reproduction in order to improve treatments for infertility and assisted reproductive technology. Her laboratory is exploring developmental benchmarks in embryos that can be reproduced and studied in model systems to improve IVF and reproductive treatments.

Inefficiencies in Human Reproduction

Compared with reproduction in other animals, human reproduction is markedly inefficient, Cook-Andersen said. The mouse cyclic fecundity rate is around 80 percent, and the nonhuman primate rate is reported to be as high as 70 percent, yet the human rate is just 20–30 percent (Silver et al., 1995; Stevens, 1997; Wilcox et al., 1988; Zinaman et al., 1996). Understanding the molecular defects in human embryo development that lead to these inefficiencies is critical to improving the diagnosis and treatment of infertility, she said. Four decades after the first IVF baby was born, observations from IVF and embryo culture in IVF clinics can provide critical insights about the most likely sources of inefficiencies in human reproduction (Steptoe and Edwards, 1978). What is learned from IVF can help to improve embryo model systems and, in turn, the embryo model systems will make it possible to understand the causes leading to these inefficiencies in our reproduction, she said. One of the major questions is precisely how IVF and embryo culture mimic what is happening in vivo. Although this question may never be fully addressed, IVF protocols provide a unique and important opportunity to observe the earliest stages of human development, Cook-Andersen said.

In humans, reproductive inefficiencies tend to occur in three different stages of embryo development, Cook-Andersen said. The first is high rates of developmental arrest: 40–50 percent of embryos arrest during the transition from the cleavage stage (day 3) to the blastocyst stage (day 5) (Hardy et al., 2001). Many of those embryos are aneuploid, but it is estimated that up to one-third of them could potentially be euploid (Maurer et al., 2015; Munné et al., 1994). For embryos that develop to the blastocyst stage, high rates of aneuploidy are a major clinical problem that is largely age-based, occurring in 25–60 percent of the embryos in women less than 40 years old and up to 90 percent of the embryos in women older than 40, she said. Even in the youngest women with the best prognoses, embryo aneuploidy rates are still as high as 20–25 percent (Franasiak et al., 2014). The third inefficiency is the high rate of implantation failure, which ranges from 30 to 70 percent per embryo transferred. Implantation failure is based partially on ploidy, but it is also related to morphology and other factors that are not yet well understood. Because these inefficiencies are more common in humans, pre-implantation developmental progression, aneuploidy and implantation are important benchmarks to study in human embryos and to reproduce in model embryo systems in order to enable the mechanistic studies required to understand the causes of these inefficiencies that cannot be performed in the embryos themselves, Cook-Andersen said.

Exploring the Molecular Basis for Successful Implantation of the Human Embryo

Cook-Andersen and her colleagues are investigating high rates of implantation failure in human embryos in order to understand ultimately what is required at the molecular level for successful implantation. Decades of studies in IVF clinics have strongly established that embryos with "good morphology" have much lower implantation failure rates and much higher live birth rates than embryos with poor morphologies (Irani et al., 2017; Nazem et al., 2019). However, the differences at the molecular level between embryos of good and poor morphology that may explain their difference in implantation potential are still unknown. Morphology is not a perfect predictor—some embryos with good morphology will not implant, and some with poor morphology will implant, Cook-Andersen said. However, her research group posits that euploid blastocysts with good morphology are enriched for embryos with high implantation potential, so euploid blastocysts with good morphology should also be enriched for the factors required for successful implantation. In the absence of being able to do rigorous genetics in humans, her laboratory is working to uncover the differences between these two groups of embryos with disparate implantation potential at the molecular level. To do this, they are exploring the gene expression patterns within and cell–cell communication networks between cells of the two major compartments of the human blastocyst: the mural trophectoderm and the inner cell mass. By directly comparing their findings in blastocysts of good and poor morphology, this approach provides the opportunity to develop prioritized gene lists and identify the molecular pathways important for successful human embryo implantation and the defects in these pathways that might contribute to the high rates of implantation failure seen in humans. Early findings suggest primitive endoderm development in pre-implantation embryos may play an important role in the success or failure of implantation, at least in the IVF setting, she said. Cook-Andersen stated that this and other similar studies in human embryos will provide important focus for studies in human embryo model systems and help lead to much needed advances in our treatments for infertile couples and in our understanding of the earliest stages of our own development.

PANEL DISCUSSION

Interactions Between Cells During Early Human Development

Discussions about human development often focus on heterogeneity and stochasticity, R. Pera said, and she asked panelists to comment about the nature of interactions that occur among cells during development (e.g., whether they are coordinated from cell to cell or are cell independent). Zernicka-Goetz replied that one of her primary research interests is to understand how an embryo breaks its symmetry with respect to the development of the major body axes and also when and how the cells within the embryo begin to differentiate and for the very first time start to initiate their identity. It is not yet known when human embryos initiate this process, but in mouse models the cells initiate this process by the four-cell stage or perhaps even earlier. The cells still have enormous plasticity potential to derive all cell lineages at that stage, Zernicka-Goetz said, albeit with different respective propensities to do so, and the potency in early blastomeres is preserved. Niakan added that disaggregating blastomeres and allowing them to develop following reaggregation has suggested that there is plasticity of cells in human embryos until even after a blastocyst is formed, but systematic lineage tracing studies to investigate this process have yet to be conducted in humans. When blastomeres are separated at the two-cell stage in the mouse, one blastomere has been recently shown to have a greater developmental potential than the other, Zernicka-Goetz said.

Naïve and Expanded-Potential Stem Cells

Panelists were asked for clarification about the definitions of naïve and expanded-potential stem cells. Earlier studies showed that ESCs can contribute to extraembryonic mesoderm, but more recent studies indicate that there is variability between naïve and expanded-potential cells. Mouse naïve cells are equivalent to epiblast at roughly 4.5 days, said Rossant. In a chimera they make epiblast derivatives but typically do not make the other cell types. Extended-potential or expanded-potential cells seem to be able to make contributions to the trophoblast. But even if they contribute to the post-implantation trophoblast, most of those cells may not necessarily be making trophoblast, although they may have further potential to make XEN and TS cells in culture, she added. In humans, these cells appear to be able to make TSCs easily, suggesting that they may have more genuinely expanded potential.

Defects in Development of Primitive Endoderm

Thus far, it appears as though the absence of the primitive endoderm signal does not affect the epiblast in terms of gene expression, but it would be expected to have an effect at later stages, said M. Pera. He asked if a similar specific defect in the extended development of primitive endoderm has been observed in embryos grown through longer stages. No specific defect in the formation of the primitive endoderm has been observed in the embryos that her laboratory has grown to post-implantation stages, Zernicka-Goetz said. However, a defect they often observe is a reduced ability of the epiblast to proliferate in vitro. She noted that specification of the epiblast and primitive endoderm occurs later in humans than in the mouse. This tissue, called hypoblast in human embryos, is essential for later development. She said that chemical signaling between the tissues is critical to maintain development of both tissues: ligands and receptors for FGF are expressed in both extraembryonic tissue and embryonic tissue, while epiblast expresses ligand. Cook-Andersen added that they have observed that the factors for those pathways were higher in good embryos than in poor ones. Her group's hypothesis is that different embryos with poor morphology might have different defects but that these different defects might all manifest similarly downstream during the development of the primitive endoderm. Some differences in gene expression can be observed in the epiblast, but they tend to be more subtle than changes in the primitive endoderm. A workshop participant suggested that single-cell databases for nonhuman primates could be analyzed for evidence of evolutionary changes that might explain the role of primitive endoderm in implantation failure in humans.

Embryo-to-Embryo Variability in Modeling Human Development

The question of how to account for embryo-to-embryo genetic and epigenetic variability in humans when translating work done using mouse models to human models was raised by a workshop participant. This variability is an important consideration and can be a confounding effect in this research, Niakan said, noting that mouse lines of certain strains also have known differences. It is difficult to work with embryos because only a fraction of them make it to the developmental stages that can be studied, she continued. Another confounding effect is that the embryos they have access to are surplus to family building (i.e., ones that were not immediately selected for IVF), so they may not be the highest quality. Some jurisdictions, such as the United Kingdom, allow the creation of embryos for research. Another option is to use surplus eggs from egg banks, which tend to have a lower maternal age of donation and may be of better quality. Zernicka-Goetz highlighted two further potential confounding factors in developing a synchronized population of human embryos to study: (1) potential mosaicism in some of the embryos and (2) determination of exactly when human embryos were activated by fertilization. The oocytes that are obtained in IVF may also be at fundamentally different developmental stages as well, R. Pera added. Obtaining a sufficient number of cells from higher-quality embryos to draw meaningful conclusions is a substantial limitation of the system, Cook-Andersen said, and another issue to consider is underlying infertility in patients, although the extent to which infertility contributes to these inefficiencies in unclear. Additionally, mosaicism and different types of aneuploidy affect large proportions of these embryos, which is a barrier to computational analysis.

Genetic and Epigenetic Aberration in Blastocysts

Suboptimal culture conditions are thought to be largely responsible for the high rate of aberration observed in embryos cultured in vitro, one workshop participant said. However, it is unclear whether naïve conditions are better or worse than standard prime conditions, the participant added. The low rate of reproductive success in humans may be due to an inherent low stability in the human system (e.g., pluripotent stem cells and certain early developmental states are transient in vivo). Potentially high rates of aberration in vivo are being "weeded out" by the biological system, but in vitro systems are being set up by selecting for cells that are compatible with culture conditions. Some data indicate that ESC lines are generally clonal, which suggests a very high selectivity for cells that may not be representative of the actual cells that contribute to reproductive success in vivo. The workshop participant went on to ask panelists if they knew of any evidence from either in vivo or in vitro cultured embryos that genetic or epigenetic aberrations may accumulate in the blastocyst itself, not in cultured cell lines where technical issues can cause aberrations. Niakan responded that more basic research is needed, but human ESC lines seem to have a high rate of acquired genomic abnormalities, such as aneuploidies or dysregulation of genes like p53, which may also underlie instability in the cells. The culture conditions for propagating human ESC and iPSC lines require optimization, Niakan said, and it would be helpful to inform approaches to optimize the culture methods by using insights from studying the embryonic compartment in the developing embryo. Due to selective pressure, embryos or cells with genomic abnormalities generally do not survive beyond a certain stage of development, Niakan said. In contrast, researchers seeking to capture these types of cells in culture in perpetuity may be selecting for a certain type of cell with slightly different properties. "This idea that you can capture exactly the equivalent stage of an embryonic transient epiblast in an in vitro culture is not necessarily an accurate way of thinking about it," Niakan said. These are useful systems for disease modeling and drug discovery, she said, but they will not always recapitulate exactly what is happening in the transient embryonic epiblast.

Future Research Directions

Panelists were asked to reflect on the research questions that emerged from the first session. Rossant commented that using stem cells to make embryo models will require answering two fundamental questions: (1) how a normal embryo develops in a human and (2) what is being captured when different stem cell states are captured. Research should be aimed at better understanding what these cells states actually are, Rossant said, rather than focusing exclusively on getting stem cells to reflect exactly what happens in the embryo. Cook-Andersen called for studies to dissect what goes wrong at each of three steps of embryo development that appear to be particularly inefficient or prone to defects. This would be valuable from a biological perspective, assuming that similar failures happen in natural development, and from a clinical perspective, because intervening to address failures during those three steps would be most beneficial for helping people with infertility. She suggested several areas of focus for future research: (1) the molecular mechanisms underpinning developmental progression on days 3–5 (which might largely reflect oocyte quality prior to fertilization); (2) the mechanisms of aneuploidy and the embryo's capacity for self-correction (including whether aneuploidy is predetermined before oocyte stimulation or if alterations in IVF stimulation protocols might decrease aneuploidy rates); and (3) the molecular requirements for successful implantation (including methods to improve embryo selection prior to transfer).

Zernicka-Goetz said that in developing their synthetic 3D models, her group drew on knowledge about mouse and human development at the time of implantation to strategically select the types and numbers of cells that are known to be involved in the epiblast, primitive endoderm, and trophectoderm at the time of implantation. This basic knowledge came from years of observations of mouse and human development before, during, and after implantation. Although synthetic models have limitations, they are a powerful resource for identifying paths of development. It would be beneficial to focus research efforts on aneuploid embryos and especially embryos that have some aneuploid cells, but many euploid cells, the so-called mosaic embryos, Zernicka-Goetz said. In the mouse, those aneuploid cells are eliminated in a part of the embryo to make the fetus, but not in trophectoderm. The elimination process peaks after implantation when the p53 pathway is initiated. If the same process is found to occur in human embryos, then the underlying mechanism could—*potentially*, she stressed—be enhanced through culturing embryos at the time of implantation. Determining the relevance of cell heterogeneity is another important research question, she said. Unlike ESCs in culture, the cells in the embryo can be homogenous before developing heterogeneity and beginning to make different structures. She suggested that this heterogeneity might help to initiate and guide this process because the embryo has limited time before it implants and must generate the three tissue types in the correct spatial-temporal order.

Niakan predicted that the advent of novel, powerful omics technologies will facilitate important comparative embryology analysis between species and help to refine hypotheses about conserved or divergent molecular programs. Furthermore, she suggested that new genome editing technologies and methods for protein depletion and manipulating gene function will contribute to identifying molecular mechanisms across species and improving stem cell biology techniques. However, she cautioned against underestimating the value of mouse and nonhuman primate models.

3

Examining the Development of Extraembryonic Lineages

Important Points Highlighted by Individual Speakers

- Using human pluripotent stem cells to model trophoblast differentiation can address the barrier of limited access to primary placenta-derived cells. (Parast)
- p63 and vestigial like family member 1 (VGLL1) are two markers of cytotrophoblast and trophoblast stem cells found in the human but not in the mouse. Further research is needed to elucidate additional key differences between mouse and human trophoblast differentiation. (Parast)
- Despite criticism of the model on various grounds, evidence shows that human embryonic stem cells treated with bone morphogenetic protein (BMP) fully differentiate to trophoblast. The BMP4/BAP-exposed cells produce a complement of hormones, including progesterone and human chorionic gonadotropin, and they express a complement of genes consistent with identity as bona fide human placental trophoblast. (Roberts)
- There are morphological, physiological, and molecular differences between primates and other mammals in early development, including the expression of chorionic gonadotropin in the human trophoblast lineage. These differences are important to consider when selecting a model to study the earliest stages of human trophoblast development. (Robson)

- RNA-sequencing approaches were used to identify specific markers (CCKBR, MRGPRX1, and syncytin-3/envP(b)) that distinguish primitive syncytium from the more mature villous trophoblast. Unlike syncytin-1 or syncytin-2, which are also expressed, syncytin-3 is abundant and specific to the primitive syncytium in late-stage human blastocysts as well as in the human embryonic stem cell–derived trophoblast. (Robson)

During the second session of the workshop, panelists explored the current state of the science about human extraembryonic lineages, including how they are defined and characterized, and they discussed the impact of extraembryonic lineages on human embryo model systems. The session was moderated by Amander Clark, a professor in and the chair of the Department of Molecular, Cell, and Developmental Biology at the University of California, Los Angeles. Clark opened the session by commenting that the talks would focus on the difficult question of what gives an embryo organismal potential.

MODELING TROPHOBLAST DIFFERENTIATION USING PLURIPOTENT STEM CELLS

Mana Parast, a professor in residence of pathology at the University of California, San Diego, presented on the use of pluripotent stem cells to model trophoblast differentiation in humans. She described trophoblast stem cells (TSCs) and the process of trophoblast differentiation, highlighting two unique markers that occur in the human but not in the mouse, and she explained how her laboratory developed their stepwise model of trophoblast differentiation. She also discussed their work in deriving TSCs from human pluripotent cells and explored the role of bone morphogenetic protein (BMP) signaling.

Trophoblast Stem Cells in Human and Mouse

Parast provided an overview of trophoblast stem cells. The concept of "pluripotent stem cell–derived trophoblast" itself is somewhat contentious, she said, because the term "totipotent" instead of "pluripotent" is usually used to characterize the cells that give rise to trophoblast (see Box 3-1). Based on data primarily from mouse models, pre-implantation inner cell mass (ICM) is thought to give rise to embryonic stem cells (ESCs) that form the embryo proper and the extraembryonic endo-

BOX 3-1
Pluripotent Versus Totipotent Stem Cells

- **Pluripotent stem cells** have the ability to give rise to embryonic cells and tissues and *some* extraembryonic cells and tissues, limited to extraembryonic endoderm and mesoderm.
- **Totipotent stem cells** have the ability to give rise to embryonic cells and tissues and to *all* extraembryonic cells/tissues, including extraembryonic endoderm, mesoderm, and ectoderm (trophoblast).

SOURCE: Mana Parast workshop presentation, January 17, 2020.

derm and mesoderm. The trophectoderm (i.e., the outer cells of the pre-implantation blastocysts) are thought to contribute only to TSCs and other trophoblast lineages. In the mouse, TSCs can be derived from pre-implantation blastocyst as well as from extraembryonic ectoderm up to embryonic day 8 (Tanaka et al., 1998). Mouse TSCs respond to fibroblast growth factor 4 (FGF4) and Activin signaling; in the absence of these factors, the cells differentiate into a combination of labyrinthine trophoblast (SynT I, SynT II, and sinusoidal giant cells) and junctional zone trophoblast (spongiotrophoblast and trophoblast giant cells). Human TSCs respond to completely different growth factors, Parast said: Wnt, epidermal growth factor (EGF), and transforming growth factor beta (TGFβ) inhibitor. Human TSCs can be derived from both blastocyst-stage embryos and early first-trimester placental tissues (Okae et al., 2018). Human TSCs are thought to be derived from the cytotrophoblast (CTB) progenitor layers, which also give rise to syncytiotrophoblast (STB) and extravillous trophoblast (EVT).

Trophoblast Differentiation

Parast went on to describe the process of trophoblast differentiation. As illustrated in Figure 3-1, the trophectoderm is believed to initially proliferate and give rise to the progenitor CTB cells. In early embryonic development, the CTB cells proliferate; these cells are primarily positive for EGF receptors as well as other markers. In anchoring villi, CTB differentiate into EVT, cells that invade the uterine tissue; they are characterized by human leukocyte antigen-G (HLA-G) expression and secrete matrix metalloproteinases (MMPs). In floating villi, CTB undergo cell–cell fusion to form STB cells that secrete human chorionic gonadotropin (hCG) and are involved

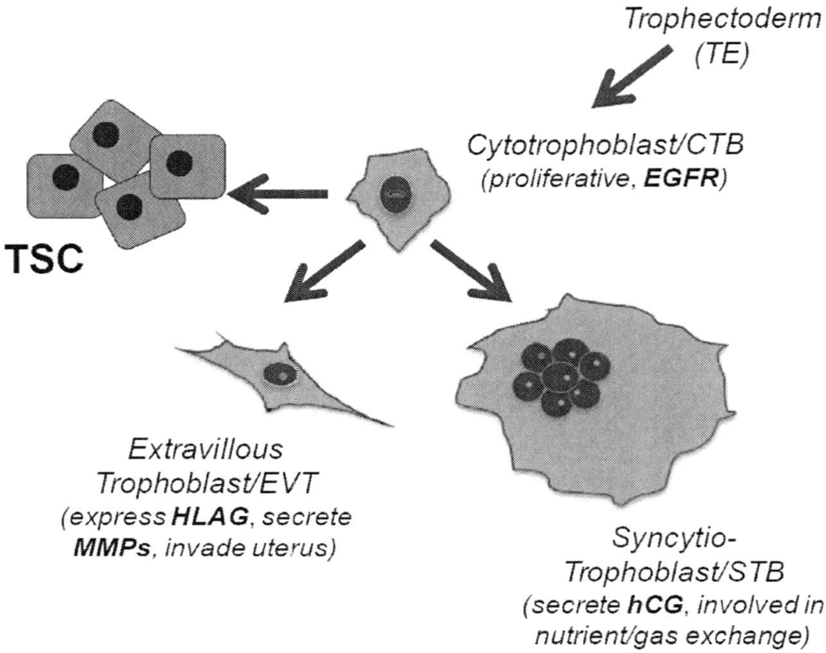

FIGURE 3-1 Human trophoblast differentiation.
NOTE: CTB = cytotrophoblast; EGFR = epidermal growth factor receptor; EVT = extravillous trophoblast; hCG = human chorionic gonadotropin; HLAG = human leukocyte antigen-G; MMP = matrix metalloproteinase; STB = syncytiotrophoblast; TE = trophectoderm; TSC = trophoblast stem cell.
SOURCE: Mana Parast workshop presentation, January 17, 2020.

in nutrient and gas exchange. The niche for TSCs is presumed to be within the CTB layer, Parast added.

Markers of Human Trophoblast Differentiation

Two specific markers of CTB and TSCs found in the human but not in the mouse were highlighted by Parast, and she noted that there are many other differences as well. The first marker is p63, a member of the p53 family of nuclear proteins that is involved in the maintenance and differentiation of stem cells in stratified epithelia (Li et al., 2013). Unlike the mouse trophoblast, the human trophoblast is organized (particularly in the villi) as a stratified epithelium with the p63-positive CTB layer being closest to the mesenchymal layer. In humans, p63 is absent in the amnion. In the human placenta, p63 expression is confined to trophoblasts, and it is expressed in all proliferative CTBs (Lee et al., 2007b). A more recently identified marker that is uniquely expressed in the human placenta is vestigial like family member 1 (VGLL1) (Soncin et al., 2018), which is a human homolog of the *Drosophila* vestigial gene that is involved in wing development. Although little is known about the function of this gene, it is known to be a binding partner for TEA domain proteins, making it a promising candidate for evaluation in the context of human trophoblast lineage specification, Parast said. Early evidence suggests that VGLL1 and TEAD4 may come together to induce p63 and trophoblast lineage in humans, much like YAP and TEAD come together to induce CDX2 and trophoblast lineage in the mouse. According to unpublished work that Parast has done with Kathy Niakan, this supposition is supported by evidence that VGLL1 and p63 are expressed in the very early trophectoderm layer of human blastocyst-stage embryos.

Modeling Human Trophoblast Differentiation

Prior to the derivation of human TSCs, models of human trophoblast differentiation were poor because the cell lines available were not fully representative of the in vivo cell type, Parast explained. Primary cells derived from the placenta are the "gold standard" in the field, but access to those cells is challenging due to issues around tissue availability. Term placentas are the most widely accessible, but term CTB can only differentiate into STB. First-trimester CTB is required to study EVT differentiation—because it can differentiate into both STB and EVT—but access to those tissues is limited and is complicated by ethical concerns. This has motivated research into the use of human pluripotent stem cells (hPSCs) to model trophoblast differentiation. One strategy used to derive trophoblast from hPSC is to culture embryoid body-derived trophoblast using 3D Matrigel (Giakoumopoulos and Golos, 2013). Another is to treat hPSC with bone morphogenetic protein 4 (BMP4) in 2D culture;[1] this strategy has been used to induce cells that resemble STB (Xu et al., 2002) as well as HLA-G-positive cells (Roberts et al., 2018).

Parast's laboratory investigates whether the treatment of human ESCs with BMP4 is a developmentally accurate model (i.e., whether the CTB cells are being obtained before the cells differentiate terminally into STB and EVT cells). Using p63 as a marker, they found that down-regulation of p63 inhibits trophoblast differentiation of human ESCs (Li et al., 2013). The cells still differentiate, but not into the terminally differentiated trophoblast that expresses HLA-G. They also observed blunted secretion of hCG and

[1]BMP4 is part of the TGFβ superfamily of proteins.

hyperglycosylated hCG. Gene expression profiling showed that the cells cluster most closely with first-trimester placental tissue and CTB rather than with other fetal and placental cells and tissues.

Developing a Stepwise Trophoblast Differentiation Model

A major criticism of the BMP-induction approach to derive CTB cells is that BMP4 is known to induce mesoderm, Parast said. However, evidence suggests BMP4 induction of mesoderm is Wnt-dependent, while BMP4 induction of trophoblast appears to be Wnt-independent (Kurek et al., 2015). Based on this finding, Parast and colleagues developed a two-step differentiation model that uses an Inhibitor of Wnt Production-2 (IWP2) in combination with BMP4 (Horii et al., 2016, 2019). Initially, this facilitates a consistent and uniform differentiation of hPSCs into CTB-like cells. A subsequent re-plating of the cells on feeder-conditioned media derives a more differentiated cell type. The advantage of this approach is that they were able to separate trophoblast lineage specification from terminal trophoblast differentiation so that the cells could be compared with primary placenta-derived CTB cells, Parast said. After the first differentiation step, Parast and her colleagues had CTB-like cells that were positive for p63, CDX2, nuclear YAP, and TEAD4. After a terminal differentiation of derived CTB cells in the second step, the majority of cells were multinucleated STB-like cells and produced hCG; 5–20 percent of the cells were EVT-like and HLA-G positive. This approach may offer an improved method to evaluate trophoblast derived from hPSCs, she said. When Parast's team compared the hPSC-derived CTB-like cells with primary CTB cells, both cell types responded to low oxygen in a similar manner (Horii et al., 2016): STB differentiation was inhibited and EVT differentiation was enhanced. Parast and her colleagues also used cells affected by trisomy 21 to demonstrate that the cells showed blunted STB differentiation that could be rescued by treatment with Activin A, just like primary CTB cells with trisomy 21.

Deriving Trophoblast Stem Cells from Human Pluripotent Cells

Another area of exploration for Parast and her colleagues involves understanding whether TSCs can be derived from human pluripotent cells. They evolved their two-step protocol by applying the media protocol used to derive human TSCs by Okae et al. (2018) to the CTB-like cells from the first step of their stepwise trophoblast differentiation model. This resulted in cells that look morphologically similar to TSCs after a few passages in the media. The cells produced by this process were positive for EGFR and found to express p63, VGLL1, GATA3, and other CTB markers. The team is currently performing ESC/trophoblast stem cell (TSC) aggregation assays to determine if the TSCs have the potential to aggregate and form embryonic-like structures. According to unpublished work by Tony Bui and Mariko Horii, an advantage of using the Okae protocol appears to be that it increases the amount of EVT-like cells by more than 80 percent, Parast said. This addresses a limitation of the second step of the previous stepwise approach, in which just 5–20 percent of the cells were EVT-like. Parast's colleagues used the updated protocol with several lines of induced pluripotent stem cells (iPSCs) derived from patients with preeclampsia. The phenotype observed using the previous two-step protocol was somewhat variable, but Bui and Horii's approach reveals a distinct phenotype between the preeclamptic and normal cell types.

BMP Signaling: Beyond Mesoderm Induction

Parast considered the role of BMP signaling beyond mesoderm induction. BMP machinery has been shown to be present in human trophectoderm (Blakeley et al., 2015). BMP signaling is also known to be required for the development of extraembryonic lineages, including trophectoderm, in the mouse pre-implantation period (Graham et al., 2014). According to unpublished work by Jennie Au and Francesca Soncin, when BMP4 is overexpressed in differentiating cultures of mouse TSCs, it blunts and inhibits differentiation. This suggests that BMP4 plays a role in the maintenance of the undifferentiated state in mouse TSCs, Parast said.

Features of Trophoblast Derived from Human Pluripotent Cells

In conclusion, Parast reflected on the question of whether hPSC-derived trophoblast cells are "real" or not. Given that the human embryo and mouse embryo develop at different rates, there may be a human-specific process by which the hESCs may not have yet undergone lineage commitment. However, BMP4 has been shown to induce some trophoblast markers in mouse ESC and mouse epiblast-derived stem cells (EpiSCs). This suggests that the process may not necessarily be human-specific, she said. As to whether it is strictly an in vitro phenomenon of "transdifferentiation," Parast countered that there may be in vivo stress conditions whereby cells derived from ESCs or EpiSCs can contribute to trophoblast. Alternatively, hPSCs or a subpopulation thereof may not even be pluripotent stem cells—they might be totipotent, because certain types of mouse ESCs have been shown to cycle between the totipotent and pluripotent state (Macfarlan et al., 2012).

NATURE OF TROPHOBLAST GENERATED FROM EMBRYONIC AND INDUCED PLURIPOTENT STEM CELLS

R. Michael Roberts, the Chancellor's Professor of animal sciences and biochemistry at the University of Missouri, examined the nature of trophoblast generated from embryonic and induced pluripotent stem cells by describing another model system that has been used to study the formation of early trophoblast from ESCs. The model uses BMP4 and inhibitors of FGF and TGFβ signaling to drive human-epiblast-type (often called "primed") ESCs and iPSCs to trophoblast. He addressed criticism that the hESCs do not fully differentiate to trophoblast in the model.

The first reported use of BMP4 to drive trophoblast formation was conducted by Xu et al. (2002), but there was also evidence in the microarray data for the presence of derivatives of both the endoderm and mesoderm and hence a mixed-lineage cell population. Further work by several groups has refined this model by excluding the factors that maintain pluripotency and including various factors that inhibit FGF2 and TGFβ/ACTIVIN signaling, which together cause the BMP4-primed cells to differentiate unidirectionally to trophoblast populations composed of both mononucleated small cells and clumps of multinucleated STB. A host of subsequent studies have used this approach to follow trophoblast emergence and the differentiation of the other sub-lineages, Roberts said.

Use of Stem Cell–Derived Trophoblasts as a Model for Placentation

Stem cell–derived trophoblasts can be used as a model for early placentation, Roberts said. The process is initiated by a brief treatment of the ESC/iPSC colonies with proteinases before cutting the colonies up into individual pieces of about 200 cells each, which are seeded into new medium, where each begins to form a new colony. The ESC/iPSC colonies are exposed to BMP4 and the FGF2 and TGFβ signaling inhibitors (the so-called BAP treatment) to drive the differentiation to trophoblast. By around day 4, uneven surfacing is evident in the colonies, a feature that becomes more extensive as culture proceeds and that reflects the emergence of STB. The cells produce increasingly larger amounts of hCG between days 6 and 8, probably reflecting the requirement for hCG production by the embryo as it implants, the need to ensure successful maternal recognition of pregnancy, and the continued production of progesterone by the maternal ovary. Earlier (days 2–6 of BAP treatment) one typically sees the emergence of cells that are HLA-G positive. These cells can invade a Matrigel matrix and move through pores in a membrane below, thereby allowing their invasiveness to be measured. Roberts emphasized that in addition to invasive features, BAP-treated hESCs clearly have a phenotype that is similar to placental trophoblast and dissimilar to any other organs and tissues. Studies of the transcriptome of BAP-treated hESC demonstrate a lack of any signature corresponding to mesoderm or other lineages except trophoblast (Jain et al., 2017). Roberts went on to outline the knowledge accumulated thus far on this BAP-treated hESC model (see Box 3-2).

Nature of BAP-Generated Trophoblast

Having established that it is not mesoderm, Roberts then spoke about the nature of this BAP-generated trophoblast, which is a focus of ongoing research. He presented a principal component analysis of transcriptomic landscapes (both single-cell and whole transcriptome) of human trophoblasts obtained from placental and tissue culture origins in order to highlight the similarities and differences between the ESC-derived trophoblast and trophoblast from other sources. He concluded that the ESC-derived cells most strongly resembled trophoblast differentiated from the trophoblast stem cells described by Okae et al. (2018).

BOX 3-2
Data Collected on the BAP-Treated hESC Model of Trophoblast Differentiation

- The BMP4/BAP-exposed cells produce a complement of hormones, including progesterone and hCG, and they express a complement of genes consistent with an identity as placental trophoblast.
- At 24 hours the cells are transiently CDX2-positive, but the CDX2 is then rapidly down-regulated; by 48 hours, all cells are KRT7-positive but largely CDX2 negative.
- HLA-G-positive CTB appear at days 2–3 and are maximal at day 6.
- Cells exhibit invasive properties.
- STB begins to form by around day 5.
- STB and CTB that are generated have distinct transcriptome profiles from villous trophoblast in terms of differentially expressed genes and microRNAs.
- The BAP-differentiated cells form organoids, or 3D multicellular tissue cultures that, in part, have characteristics resembling those of an organ.

SOURCE: R. Michael Roberts workshop presentation, January 17, 2020.

Dynamics of Early Trophoblast Development in Cultured Human Embryos

To frame his discussion of the dynamics of early trophoblast development in cultured human embryos, Roberts sketched the early stages of human placental development. The early stages of implantation are associated with the formation of an invasive STB that "burrows" into the endometrium. He suggested that BAP-differentiated cells correspond most closely to this syncytial mass associated with embryo implantation rather than to the STB associated with either mature placental villi or even the little understood, multi-nuclear trophoblast giant cells embedded deep in the endometrium (Turco and Moffett, 2019). However, some unique markers are shared between ESC-generated trophoblast and the STB associated with early placental villi during the early weeks of the first trimester of a human pregnancy.

Roberts then described a single-cell RNAseq analysis performed on cultured human blastocysts, which, between days 8 and 12 of culture, appear to develop much as they appear to do in vivo, including forming an outer shell of STB and producing large amounts of hCG (West et al., 2019). By showing a live cell microscopy movie during the workshop, Roberts demonstrated the materialization of a hitherto unknown, migratory trophoblast cell around embryonic day 10 that moves away from the embryo. These cells are positive for HLA-G and share some markers with the extravillous trophoblast cells that later in placental development invade the endometrium from the tips of anchoring placental villi. The single-cell RNAseq analysis also revealed how proliferating cytotrophoblast closer to the embryo proper give rise to two more differentiated populations of cytotrophoblast, one with some of the markers defining the motile cells, and the other carrying some STB markers shared by the large STB cells (West et al., 2019). Roberts concluded that the BAP-differentiated trophoblast generated from ESCs and iPSCs might provide ideal models for studying these early stages of human pregnancy without using human embryos.

"Failed" Criteria for ESC-Derived Trophoblast

The BAP model has been criticized on various grounds, Roberts said (Lee et al., 2016). One line of criticism is that the ELF5 promoter in the differentiating cells remains hypermethylated; however, this is perhaps not surprising because early human trophoblast appears not to express the *ELF5* gene extensively, if at all. Another criticism is the lack of expression of C19-encoded miRNA; Roberts conceded that the ESCs down-regulate this locus as they differentiate, but it is unclear what this means. However, he rebutted the criticism that ESC-derived trophoblast do not express HLA-G and have an uncharacteristic HLA profile. All papers where an adequate analysis was performed have revealed robust production of HLA-G and the full-length HLA-G transcript, he said. The perceived lack of positive trophoblast markers is also unquestionably wrong. In conclusion, Roberts maintained that BAP-treated human ESCs fully differentiate to trophoblast, although that trophoblast is different from that associated with villous trophoblast later in pregnancy.

Roberts added that there are several potential uses of trophoblast generated from ESCs and iPSCs, in addition to studying early trophoblast differentiation. These potential uses include (1) assessing toxicology and responses to foreign agents, (2) generating TSCs, (3) following trophoblast lineage divergence, (4) studying origins of placental disease (e.g., preeclampsia), and (5) evaluating the susceptibility of early trophoblast to pathogens (e.g., Zika virus) (Sheridan et al., 2018, 2019; Yang et al., 2015).

MOLECULAR INNOVATION IN THE HUMAN TROPHOBLAST LINEAGE

Paul Robson, an associate professor and the director of single-cell biology at The Jackson Laboratory in Farmington, Connecticut, discussed molecular evolutionary innovation in the human trophoblast lineage. He noted that Parast and Roberts provided evidence that it is possible to get trophoblast from pluripotent cells and that these models provide an opportunity to look at the earliest states of human trophoblast. In his presentation he emphasized the molecular differences between species by focusing on work that uses those models to study the cells' molecular features and uses comparative genomics to look at the sequences that are functional in these cells.

Variation in Early Development Across Species

Robson opened by explaining the concept of conservation of evolution and development. As reflected in the "hourglass" model, it is thought that species-to-species differences in the developing organisms are most pronounced early in development and late in development, with the conserved part of development in the phylotypic stage (Kalinka and Tomancak, 2012) (see Figure 3-2). The phylotypic stage occurs much later in development than the blastocyst: in the human, it occurs 4 weeks post-fertilization; in the mouse, it occurs about 10 days post-fertilization. Based on the hourglass model, significant differences would be expected in comparative embryology.

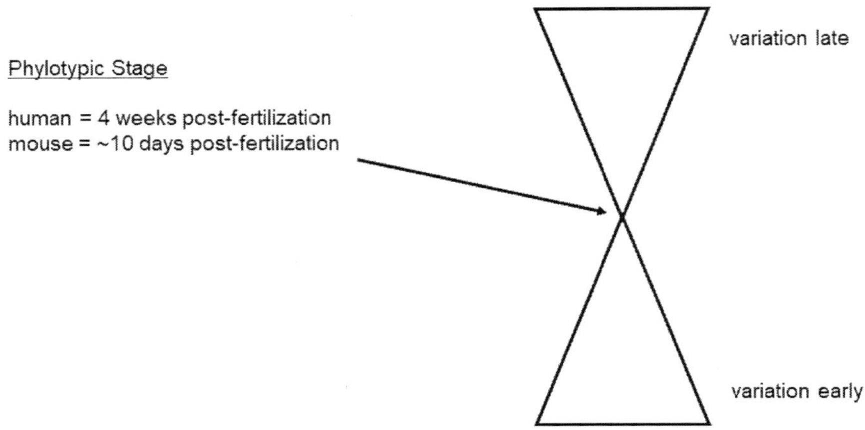

FIGURE 3-2 The hourglass model of variation in early development.
SOURCE: Paul Robson workshop presentation, January 17, 2020.

Differences Between Primates and Other Mammals in Early Development

Robson explored some of the morphological, physiological, and molecular differences between primates and other mammals in early development, noting that different features of human versus mouse embryology are well established and had been discussed by other speakers. Morphological differences between primates have been demonstrated by a cladistic analysis of the ontogeny of primate fetal membranes, which positions species accurately in the phylogenetic tree based on differential features in early embryonic development (Luckett, 1976). This type of analysis elucidates differences not only between the mouse and the human, but also between the human and old-world monkeys, for example.

Physiological and Molecular Differences Between Simians and Other Mammals

Substantial physiological differences are also evident between simians and other mammals during this early period of development, Robson said. A simian-specific feature of this developmental time period is that the endometrium goes through spontaneous decidualization[2] and menstruation.

[2]Decidualization refers to the process of rapid proliferation and differentiation of endometrial stromal cells into decidual cells, which is required for implantation (Haller et al., 2019).

Therefore, the implanting blastocyst is intimately interacting with this simian-specific feature of endometrial tissue. This difference motivated the working hypothesis that the primitive syncytium co-evolved with spontaneous decidualization and menstruation because it attaches, invades, and embeds in the endometrium.

Evidence also shows significant molecular differences hardwired in the genome that underpin these physiological and morphological differences, Robson said. To illustrate, he offered the example of a newly evolved system for hCG, an essential hormone for pregnancy that is simian-specific; hCG must be expressed in the implanting embryo, or the embryo will be immediately aborted. Chorionic gonadotropin (CG) is expressed by the late-stage human blastocyst and the syncytium. The CG signal is required to block menstruation; thus, it is essential to maintain pregnancy. CG is derived from anterior pituitary hormones (specifically luteinizing hormone) that went through a gene duplication 40 million years ago to form the beta peptide of chorionic gonadotropin (CGB). Both the alpha peptide (CGA) and CGB of hCG had to evolve the regulatory architecture to be expressed in the trophoblast lineage. These molecules are not expressed in the mouse trophoblast, although paralogs are expressed in the anterior pituitary.

Transgenic mice have been used to study the regulation of human CGA, Robson said. This work found that anterior pituitary expression was faithfully maintained in the mice, but there was no expression in the mouse trophoblast, suggesting that there are transcription factors in the human trophoblast that are not present in the mouse trophoblast to drive expression of this gene. This highly specific expression of CGA in the mouse system is only in the anterior pituitary. He noted that in one of the early publications on mouse epiblast stem cells treated with BMP4, one of the four genes used to try to establish similarities between mouse and human ESCs was CGA (Brons et al., 2007).

Molecular Signature of Primitive Syncytium Evident in Late-Stage Human Blastocyst

To characterize the molecular signature of the primitive syncytium, Robson and colleagues generated single-embryo RNA-sequencing data through pre-implantation development. In the 7-day blastocyst they found a signature that is clearly indicative of a syncytial cell signature. It includes the glial cells missing transcription factor 1 (GCM1)—the "master regulator" of syncytialization—as well as syncytin itself and other genes in the estrogen biosynthetic pathway (e.g., HSD3B1). This signature equates with the CCR7/GCM1+ polar trophectoderm population defined in Petropoulos et al. (2016). Robson explained that because these genes are not found in the mouse blastocyst, this work clearly indicates the emergence of the syncytial transcriptome in the late-stage human blastocyst. This fits with the corpus of existing morphological studies, because the syncytial cell forms as soon as the human embryo implants. This model, or variations thereof, has been used extensively to show that hESC treated with BMP4 and FGF inhibitor result in blastocycstic trophoblast and primitive syncytium, Robson said (Xu et al., 2002; Yabe et al., 2016). Studies measuring the transcriptional response to BMP4 using ChIP-seq experiments clearly demonstrate that trophectoderm transcription factors are direct targets of BMP4. Classic trophoblast transcription factors such as GATA2, GATA3, and AP2A all have SMAD1/5/8 binding sites and immediately upregulate upon BMP4 induction, which explains how trophoblast is being driven from ESCs.

Markers of Primitive Syncytium Derived from Human Embryonic Stem Cells

Robson highlighted several markers of hESC-derived primitive syncytium established by RNA-sequencing data comparing the human villous placenta (i.e., later-stage trophoblast) to hESC-derived trophoblast and to the late-stage blastocyst. Although there are many similarities between the primitive syncytium and the villous STB, the specific markers that distinguish primitive syncytium from the more mature villous trophoblast include CCKBR, MRGPRX1, and syncytin-3/envP(b). He noted that unlike syncytin-1 or syncytin-2, which are also expressed, syncytin-3 is abundant and fairly specific to this primitive syncytium in the late-stage blastocysts as well as in the human ESC-derived trophoblast; it is much lower in the villous trophoblast. Thus, syncytin-3 is another example of a simian-specific trophoblast gene that has been co-opted from an endogenous retrovirus insertion 40 million years ago. Another example is the co-option of a long-terminal repeat to drive *CYP19A1* expression in the human trophoblast, contributing to the activity of the estrogen biosynthetic pathway from dehydroepiandrosterone sulfate (DHEA-S) to estrogen production; this pathway is known to be active in the human placenta, but not the mouse placenta. It is also active in the primitive syncytium derived from pluripotent cells. Robson suggested that DHEA-S-derived estrogen production is a useful functional assay for the primitive syncytium or any human syncytiotrophoblast. Adding DHEA or DHEA-S to the trophoblast medium results in large amounts of estrogen being produced, which indicates that the biochemical pathway is active.

Molecular Heterochrony in a Developmental Regulator: GCM1

To look more deeply at molecular control of the primitive syncytium, Robson returned to GCM1, the classic master regulator of syncytial formation. GCM1 has been knocked out in the mouse and is lethal to the embryo until embryonic days 8.5–9, which is when the syncytium forms in the mouse placenta, at a much later developmental stage than in humans. It has also been characterized in human placental explants, and it is functionally involved in syncytialization of the villous. Because it is expressed in the human at the blastocyst stage, which is much earlier than in the mouse, there is interest in characterizing it further. CRISPR technologies have been used to knock it out in iPSCs and to conduct gene expression using pluripotent cell differentiation protocols; when this is done, it drastically reduces syncytialization, as anticipated. However, global gene expression techniques reveal large numbers of altered genes and the apparent upregulation of CTB markers. Robson said that some of the top GCM1-bound and functional cis regulatory elements within PSC-derived trophoblast have emerged over recent evolutionary time.

Robson provided two examples of GCM1 target genes in the primitive syncytium: LMO2 and ALX4. In humans the LMO2 proximal promoter contains five GCM1 binding sites. However, the binding sites have been lost in other species, with no evidence for GCM1 cis regulatory elements in the mouse, for example. ALX4 is a similar example of a GCM1 target gene in the primitive syncytium. This gene is down-regulated in the GCM1 knockout, so it is a functional binding site. As with LMO2, there are species-specific differences that are indicative of active evolutionary change around the regulatory regions that bind GCM1 and drive expression of these transcriptional regulators in primitive syncytium.

Early Development as a Site for Rapid Mutation and Selection

Robson concluded by emphasizing the extent of the molecular and functional differences between species in the primitive syncytium and predicting that there are significant differences in other cell types at these early stages of development. He surmised that this period of early development is a window of rapid selection and mutation in the human population. Therefore, he suggested altering the hourglass model to increase the size at the bottom of the hourglass, because there is probably much more variation early in development than in later development. He added that early development probably creates selection pressure for many novelties as humans and other species evolve. In fact, there may be variation of the human population being selected for today. If selection is occurring early in development (e.g., aborting an embryo that is dysfunctional at 4 weeks, rather than leading to likely death at 25 years in an adult) it allows for an increased rate of evolution. For instance, the single-nucleotide polymorphism (SNP) in the human population that appears to be most strongly selected for is a SNP in EPAS1, the gene encoding HIF2-alpha. It appears to have been rapidly selected for among Tibetans, presumably through the low-oxygen environment at high altitude, as this is an oxygen-sensing transcription factor. Some have suggested that it regulates oxygen concentration in adults, allowing them to live more comfortably at high altitudes. It is also well known that oxygen sensing is an important feature of trophoblast development. Of note, the lineage decision between a CTB and an STB is oxygen-regulated, and EPAS1 is the most highly abundant transcription factor expressed in these hESC-derived primitive syncytial cells.

PANEL DISCUSSION

Variability in Trophoblast-Related Terminology

Panelists were asked by Amander Clark, the session moderator, to explain why they refer to the trophoblast system as a syncytium and how that relates to the syncytiotrophoblast, CTB, mural trophoblast, or polar trophoblast. She also asked how the primitive syncytium relates to the cell types differentiated in their pluripotent stem cell models.

The terminology can be confusing, Roberts said. It was initially presumed that the syncytium that was forming was villous STB, but it later became clear that it was not. Others have claimed that it is mesoderm, but the question of what it actually is remains open. Roberts uses the term "primitive placenta," because it represents the placenta's function very early in development when it is developing at the expense of locally produced histrophe and attempting to produce sufficient hormones to maintain the pregnancy. The trophoblast is a complex lineage of cells with multiple subtypes, Robson replied, which gives rise to definitional challenges. Many studies have compared the pluripotent cell–derived trophoblast to villous trophoblast because it is accessible, but it comes from the placenta much later in development (7–8 weeks) and its composition is completely different. Robson characterized this as a progression: the trophoblast in the peri-implantation stage that he described in his presentation—the blastocystic trophoblast—is the first trophoblast which seals the blastocyst. The next apparent trophoblast is the primitive syncytium, a term first established in the 1960s (Boyd and Hamilton, 1966). The use of terminology in this work is variable across the disciplines of cell and developmental biology, placental researchers, and pathologists, Parast said. Efforts have been made to standardize definitions, but in the case of primitive syncytium this is challenging because the nature of the cell is still unknown. Presumably, the cell has a combination of characteristics from the STB (e.g., it is multinucleated and expresses some of the factors that induce cell–cell fusion) while also having invasive potential. There is still much to learn about the primary cell types using the embryo and the placenta to determine the nature of the cells in culture, Parast said.

Differentiation of Trophoblast Versus Amnion Cell Lineages

A workshop participant commented that recent self-organizing models have shown the development of amnion is dependent on BMP. Given that there are many markers shared by amnion and trophoblast and that the emergence of amnion from the epiblast is more aligned with what is thought to occur during early development in vivo, the participant asked the panelists to comment on the relationship between their models and amnion differentiation. He also asked about the molecular pathways that may turn cells to trophoblast versus amnion lineages. p63 is not expressed in the amnion and is not required for amniogenesis, Parast said, because p63-null mice survive through embryogenesis. Furthermore, the initial burst of transcription factor, Brachyury, occurs when amnion is generated and does not occur during trophoblast differentiation, particularly in the presence of IWP2. A challenge is that there is currently no measurement of real amnion formation in humans, Robson said. He suggested that the absence of Brachyury expression suggests that BMP4 and FGF inhibition are directly up-regulating classic trophoblast markers. BMP is involved in multiple differentiation pathways, so it could potentially play a role in both amnion and trophoblast systems. Roberts maintained that there is no evidence that amnion produces any of these characteristic trophoblast products.

Cells Used to Direct Trophoblast Stem Cell Derivation

A workshop participant asked Parast whether the protocol she follows to direct TSC derivation used undirected pluripotent cells or BMP-derived cells. She replied the cells were already BMP-derived cells at the end of the first step. After a 4-day differentiation in the presence of BMP4 and IWP2, they switch to the Okae media for several passages. In the original Okae study, the TSCs were derived from trophectoderm of blastocyst-stage embryos as well as from early placenta villous CTB. The participant inquired about detailed molecular analysis of what the PSC-derived trophoblasts are being reverted to; Parast replied that the RNA-sequencing data will be available soon.

Syncytin-3 Expression

A workshop participant requested clarification on the identity of syncytin-3 and how it relates to the other syncytins. Syncytin-3 is in the intron of the gene Rin3, Robson said, and it is a 40-million-year-old simian-specific insertion, so it is the same age as syncytin-2. It is immunogenic and fusogenic, according to functional studies in cell lines conducted when it was first identified by virologists (Blaise et al., 2005). Robson and colleagues found that it is significantly expressed both in the late blastocyst and in primitive syncytium derived from ESCs.

Heterogeneity in Trophectoderm

The topic of heterogeneity in the trophectoderm during the transition from pre-implantation to peri-implantation was raised by a workshop participant. The publication by Petropoulos et al. (2016) clearly shows heterogeneity and indicates a transition in trophectoderm closest to embryo (i.e., polar cells), Roberts said. This developmental progression coincides both with implantation and likely with the emergence of invasive syncytium from those cells. In the blastocyst it is not syncytial, but it becomes syncytial as it implants. Robson added that primitive syncytium probably forms at the polar end of the human blastocyst upon attachment. Parast noted that this heterogeneity also extends to post-implantation CTB. Single-cell sequencing of placental tissues at 5–7 weeks reveals multiple cell populations in the CTB that seem to differ according to their proximity to the fetal versus maternal surfaces.

Wnt Signaling in Trophectoderm

The function of Wnt signaling in the trophectoderm was raised by a workshop participant. Parast and colleagues are using Wnt inhibition to get from the pluripotent state to the CTB state; it appears that this may limit BMP4-induced mesoderm induction. In the trophectoderm itself, Wnt signaling seems to be important in maintaining the undifferentiated state, Parast said, but its role is complicated. Wnt has to be withdrawn to initiate differentiation into extravillous trophoblast, then Wnt has to be re-added to get full differentiation into mature extravillous trophoblast (Haider et al., 2018).

Trophoblast in the Peri-Implantation Window

The panelists were asked to reflect on the trophoblast in the peri-implantation window and the various differentiation approaches that are or could be used to make trophoblast from stem cells. Robson's laboratory is deriving trophoblast directly from human ESCs. Because ESCs are also used to model other definitive lineages, he suggested that a novel strategy could be devised to derive both trophoblast and the other lineages simultaneously in the same structure. Parast suggested further exploring the mouse system to generate chimeras and examine contributions to trophectoderm, given the ethical challenges of working with human and nonhuman primate models. Roberts argued that the current model is totally unsatisfactory and needs to be refined. For example, markers observed in trophoblast are not observed even in the early embryo; the function of BMP4 is also unknown. Further mouse research will be needed to understand and improve the system, he said. The embryo does not develop in isolation, Robson noted. Cross-communication between the embryo and endometrium—in addition to bidirectional signaling from the syncytium—is likely informing developmental decisions in ways that are not yet understood. Organoid systems are available to study the human endometrium, and co-culturing PSC-derived cells with these will be important, he said.

Role of Trophoblast Signaling in Inducing Gastrulation

The panelists were asked whether early human trophoblast must signal to the epiblast to induce the processes of gastrulation, given that (1) in humans the first trophoblast develops as primary syncytium and (2) in the mouse, signals from the primitive endoderm and signals between epiblast and trophoblast are critical for early patterning. Parast replied that they are investigating this crosstalk between trophoblast and other cells by co-culturing human ESCs and TSCs, and it looks as though ESCs remain relatively undifferentiated, at least morphologically.

4

Stem Cell–Based Models of Human Embryos

Important Points Highlighted by Individual Speakers

- The scarcity of biological material (e.g., human in vitro fertilization embryos) for studying early human embryonic development is a barrier to clinical breakthroughs and biomedical discovery, and stem cell–based models of human embryos can be useful in conducting this work. (Brivanlou, Rivron)
- Geometrically confining human embryonic stem cells and adding a single growth factor (bone morphogenetic protein 4) causes the cells to self-organize into gastruloids with all three germ layers through mechanisms of edge sensing and reaction diffusion. Gastruloids are a valuable model system because they allow for quantitative analysis and cellular responses can be tracked at a single-cell resolution. (Brivanlou, Warmflash)
- Recent studies of gastruloids suggest that Huntington's disease is actually a developmental condition, not a neurodegenerative one. Further work on gastruloids holds great promise for modeling and potentially treating human diseases. (Brivanlou)
- Compared with in vivo systems, synthetic embryology provides a wealth of opportunities to understand how cells differentiate, self-organize, regulate each other, and propagate through a colony over time. (Warmflash)

- Single-cell RNA sequencing of gastruloids can reveal novel human-specific molecular signatures, such as yolk sac trophectoderm. (Brivanlou)
- Embryo models can be generated in large numbers and are conducive to gene editing, providing a platform for high-throughput genetic and drug screens. (Rivron)
- The aim of synthetic embryology is to answer specific questions about early human embryo development using systems that mimic specific certain features of cell patterning, signal dynamics, and molecular mechanisms. The aim of synthetic embryology is not to build actual embryos from stem cells—in fact, these systems fail to break symmetry and lack organismal potential to develop further if they are implanted. (Warmflash)
- In three-dimensional (3D) culture conditions, trophoblast stem cells and embryonic stem cells can self-organize to generate blastocyst-like structures (blastoids) that recapitulate specific aspects of implantation and early development in utero, but do not have organismal potential. (Rivron)
- Trophospheres can be generated using the same process as blastoids, but without the presence of organic cells. Comparing trophospheres to blastoids reveals that embryonic inductions are important in inducing trophoblast proliferation and self-renewal as well as in preparing them for implantation in the uterus. (Rivron)
- Microfluidic systems can be used to model features of peri-implantation human development using human pluripotent stem cells—such as self-organization into multicellular structures, lumenogenesis, and even differentiation into amniotic ectoderm-like cells—which enables research on cell signaling dynamics, signaling propagation, and inductive signals that drive the formation of different compartments. Microfluidic systems appear to be more controllable and reproducible than the conventional 3D culture environment. (Fu)

The third session of the workshop centered on models of the human embryo based on stem cells. Panelists described the latest scientific and technical developments with models of human embryos and considered directions for future research and applications of this work. They also examined the fidelity of human embryo model systems to bona fide human embryos and explored methods for validation of the model systems. The session was moderated by Arnold Kriegstein, a professor of neurology and the director of the developmental and stem cell biology program at the University of California, San Francisco.

GASTRULOIDS: MODELING HUMAN EMBRYOS AND EMBRYONIC TISSUES

Ali Brivanlou, the Robert and Harriet Heilbrunn Professor at The Rockefeller University, introduced synthetic self-organizing models of human embryos called "gastruloids" and highlighted lessons about the basic science of human development that can be gleaned from these models. From a utilitarian perspective, he also made the case for the use of synthetic models as a tool for addressing diseases whose roots can be traced to very early human embryonic development. He began by describing the rationale for human embryological studies more broadly (see Box 4-1).

In Vitro Attachment and Self-Organization in Early Human Embryonic Development

Brivanlou opened by presenting a series of images to trace the development of the embryo over the first 2 weeks of development, noting that very few pictures are available that represent this early developmental

BOX 4-1
Rationale for Human Embryological Studies

- Understanding of our own human origins;
- Investigating species-specific molecular and cellular differences that cannot be studied in model systems;
- Improving reproductive medicine and understanding why more than half of natural human blastocysts fail to implant; and
- Developing therapies for developmental diseases.

SOURCE: Ali Brivanlou workshop presentation, January 17, 2020.

stage. At day 8, the in vitro attached human embryo displays an amazing ability to self-organize in radially symmetrical patterns. The inner cell mass (ICM) can be observed with the trophectoderm around it. He said that his assumption had been that as soon as the embryo attaches, inductive interactions between maternal tissue and embryonic tissue would be required for the proper induction and patterning of cell fate, so observing this happening independently without apparent extrinsic influences was unexpected for him. At day 12, this self-organization continues to progress, with increasingly aesthetically attractive attributes. He highlighted the ratio between trophectoderm and the ICM at day 10 and then at day 12, noting that a large fraction of the attached embryos lack epiblast cells. Again, he emphasized the aesthetic features of this self-organization: the cells are radially patterned, and the yolk sac and amniotic cavity are nicely proportioned with similar numbers of cells.

Rationale for Human Embryo Models

Motivated by these types of observations about in vitro attachment and self-organization in early human embryonic development, Brivanlou and colleagues began exploring the extent to which knowledge gained from model systems is valid in humans by investigating whether these types of attributes are (1) human-specific or (2) attributes that have been evolutionarily conserved. In exploring these questions, they were able to detect human biological features that had never before been identified in the embryo of any other mammalian species. For example, they discovered the novel human cell type yolk sac trophectoderm (ysTE), which has a unique molecular signature ($OCT4^{LO}$ $GATA6^{LO}$ $GATA3^{+}$ $CDX2^{+}$) never before seen in any other mammalian embryo (Deglincerti et al., 2016; Zhou et al., 2019). This type of discovery underscores the importance of working with human tissue, he said.

Brivanlou delved further into the rationale for studying human embryo models—"gastruloids"—that are derived from human embryonic stem cells (hESCs) (Warmflash et al., 2014). One reason for using human embryo models is the 14-day limit.[1] However, even in the absence of such a guideline, there will never be sufficient sources of biological material available to thoroughly investigate our human origins, such as the molecular basis of human cell pattern formation and the emergence of organs and the tissues, Brivanlou said. Surmounting this barrier will require developing model systems that can provide the large numbers of biological samples that are required to conduct this work. Mouse models and nonhuman primate

[1]The 14-day rule refers to a policy that restricts the culture of human embryos past 14 days of development.

models have value, he said, but making meaningful progress will require exploring species-specific facets of development with human models. From a utilitarian perspective, clinical breakthroughs are dependent on this type of research, particularly the development of therapies for diseases with a developmental origin and especially for those diseases that develop after the 14-day point. Model human embryos can facilitate those types of clinical breakthroughs for diseases that affect the early embryo or fetus—which he characterized as long overdue—without the need for human embryos. "The only way to move forward where that system has mostly failed us is to bite the bullet and move forward with human studies," Brivanlou said.

Creating Model Human Gastruloids Derived from Human Embryonic Stem Cells

Brivanlou described how these model human gastruloids are created using hESCs. When the hESCs are cultured under standard conditions, the variations in size and density of colonies—some colonies are touching other colonies, some colonies are completely independent of one another—and the presence of individual randomly dispersed cells make it impossible to replicate the system and quantify it at a subcellular level. This may be a reason why different laboratories performing the same experiment generate inconsistent results under identical experimental conditions, he noted. To address this issue, Aryeh Warmflash, who would speak next in the session, created a process for imposing a standard on hESCs by developing micropattern technology whereby the hESCs would only adhere to a circular substrate (85–1,000 microns in size) (Warmflash et al., 2014). At a minimum, this allows for imposing size and dimension homogeneity in the culture, with the potential to bring in more quantitative approaches as well. Warmflash and colleagues also developed the programming technology to track and evaluate single-cell resolution response to a given stimuli. When this process is performed over thousands of cells and hundreds of colonies, cell behaviors can be measured in a way that is highly reproducible. This technology has moved forward in Brivanlou's laboratory, where they are applying deep neural networks and artificial intelligence to track the behavior of these cells.

Self-Organization of hESCs into Gastruloids by Geometrical Confinement in Response to Bone Morphogenetic Protein 4

Brivanlou described a seminal result of those first experiments with geometrical confinement (Warmflash et al., 2014). When the hESC colony maintained in pluripotency media was stimulated only with BMP4 for 48 hours, the result was dramatic. The hESC colony self-organized into gastruloids containing ectoderm (SOX2), mesoderm (BRACHYURY, or BRA), and trophectoderm (CDX2). This can be reproduced over many thousands of colonies with exactly the same precision. Brivanlou maintained that this process of geometrical confinement settles any debate over whether bone morphogenetic protein 4 (BMP4) induces trophectoderm or mesoderm. Geometrical confinement is sufficient to give rise to all the cell types in response to a single stimulus. "Confinement of geometry ... can induce everything as long as you give it an edge," he said. This holds true not only for ectoderm, mesoderm, and extraembryonic tissue, but also for endoderm (SOX17), primitive streak (zinc finger protein SNAI1, or SNAIL), and primordial germ cells (B-lymphocyte-induced maturation protein 1, or BLIMP1). The embryo contains no cell type that does not self-organize in this type of symmetry, he added. He explained that this powerful tool has enabled new avenues of research into how cell fate is established in these self-organizing patterns. It also eliminates the challenge of embryo-to-embryo variation because the process creates homogeneity not only in size, density, and cell number, but also in the cells' genotypes.

Lessons from Studying Human Gastruloids

Brivanlou highlighted several lessons learned by studying human gastruloids that would be impossible to glean from studying human embryos within the current guidelines. The first is that gastruloids self-organize through mechanisms of edge sensing and reaction diffusion (Etoc et al., 2016). Cells establish their fate in these circular colonies by measuring their distance from the edge, he explained. This can be demonstrated with various techniques, including the use of CRISPR/Cas9, to show that the wave of transcriptional response patterning starts from the edge and moves inward to crash in the center (i.e., the reverse of throwing a pebble in water). The second lesson is that Wnt signaling memory is required for Activin to function as a morphogen (Yoney et al., 2018). History matters for cells' fate, Brivanlou explained. A cell knows who it is in the gastruloid based on the history of signaling it has been exposed to. This could not have been learned without manipulating the sequence in which the ligand stimulus is presented at different times. The third lesson is that a wave of Wnt signaling controls primitive streak formation downstream of the BMP4 signaling, which can be functionally demonstrated using grafting in a chick embryo (Martyn et al., 2019). Single-cell RNA sequencing of gastruloids can reveal novel human-specific molecular signatures, he said. For example, his laboratory has recently discovered a group of genes in humans that have never before been associated with primordial germ cells. Among the most unexpected was DOCK2, a gene that previously was associated only with the migration of white blood cells and lymphocytes from the blood cells out to the target. This finding suggests that the early migration of primordial germ cells in humans follows pathways and molecular hierarchies that are already known, he said, which creates the potential for developing interventions in the future.

Near Horizon: Three-Dimensional Gastruloids and Symmetry Breaking

The two-dimensional (2D) embryo modeling systems are useful, Brivanlou said, but the human embryo is three dimensional (3D). Fortunately, a generation of 3D gastruloids that undergo symmetry breaking is on the near horizon. A method has already been developed to change substrate stiffness in 3D colonies to generate what looks like primitive endoderm (GATA6) and trophectoderm (GATA3) (Deglincerti et al., 2016; Simunovic et al., 2019). The method involves dissociating the cells and combining them with a 3D epiblast grown in a combination of Matrigel and hydrogel. High-fidelity modeling is then used to monitor the development. At day 1 post-mixing, the geometries of epiblast, amniotic cavity, and yolk sac cavity that emerge in the in vitro attached embryo appear similar to embryos developed in vivo. After 3 days, the phenomenon of symmetry breaking—indicated by GATA3, BRA, and SOX2—was observed in the self-organizing 3D embryos. Work is under way to validate this model by comparing 3D embryos to real embryos attached in vitro at day 8, he said. Morphologically they appear similar; their molecular signatures indicate that they are close but not identical. Single-cell RNA sequencing is in progress to compare the specimens and evaluate the similarities and differences between their respective cell types in the hope that new cell types might be identified.[2]

Modeling Human Disease in Gastruloids and Neuruloids

In the final part of his presentation, Brivanlou commented on the application of human embryo models to cure human diseases. This utilitarian aspect is important to consider, particularly in the context of using public funding, he said. To explore whether diseases can be modeled in gastruloids, his laboratory decided to target Huntington's disease. It is relatively straightforward to investigate because it is caused by a single dominant mutation in the HTT gene.[3] It is considered to be a neuro-

[2]Brivanlou noted that the ysTE discovered in the attached human embryo does not exist in the model embryo, which is a positive finding.

[3]The mutation that results in Huntington's disease causes a polyglutamine (polyQ) expansion in the HTT protein.

degenerative disease and currently has no therapy or cure. Despite the fact that it was the first gene cloned with 100 percent penetrance for the state of the disease, model systems have failed to accurately replicate the disease thus far. The discovery of an isoform of Huntington's disease only present and expressed in hominids—but not marmosets or lower primates—suggests that the reliance on mouse or lower nonhuman primate models may be a reason that the model systems have failed (Ruzo et al., 2018). That is, they may have been working with systems that do not represent the molecular signature of the target disease. To investigate, Brivanlou's laboratory generated a series of isogenic human ESC lines to introduce the Huntington's disease mutation in gastruloids. Immediately it created a phenotypic signature that was also dependent on the length of the repeating CAG (cytosine-adenine-guanine) section segment in the gene (i.e., gastruloids with different insertions displayed related but different phenotypes). This finding suggested for the first time that Huntington's disease is actually a developmental disease, not a neurodegenerative disease. The center section of gastruloids can be used to generate another type of self-organizing structure called neuruloids, which can also be used to model Huntington's disease. Neuruloids are self-organizing ectodermal structures that display radial distribution of cell types, with brain cells at the center, surrounded by neural crest and neural placodes (sensory organs) and epidermis covering the entire structure. Neuruloids also display a specific phenotypic signature for Huntington's disease. The researchers are now selecting for compounds that can rescue the phenotype from the neuruloid and gastruloid back to the non-Huntington's disease phenotype. High-throughput screening has identified five compounds that can rescue the phenotypes seen in Huntington neuruloids, and the researchers are ready to move to the next stage of medicinal chemistry. Brivanlou added that similar disease modeling is in progress for fragile X (FMR1), tuberous sclerosis (TSC1 and 2), and autism (MECP2). Because neuruloids can be pushed to self-organized circuitry, they are being used to look at psychiatric diseases and circuitries in different tissues and organs. Another line of research is using these models to look at infectious diseases such as Zika virus, HIV, and cytomegalovirus 1, in which the fetal and early embryo are known targets of the viral infection.

MODELING HUMAN DEVELOPMENT IN 2D WITH MICROPATTERNS

Aryeh Warmflash, a principal investigator and an assistant professor in the Department of Biosciences at Rice University, discussed how human development can be modeled in 2D using micropatterns. He offered insights into how gastruloid systems generate patterns and considered ways forward to generate models that can help to answer specific developmental questions.

Geometric Confinement Triggers Self-Organized Patterning Along the Colony Axis

As Brivanlou described, Warmflash and his colleagues found that by geometrically confining human ESCs and adding a single growth factor, BMP4, the cells self-organize into trophectoderm-type cells with all three germ layers—endoderm, mesoderm, and ectoderm (Warmflash et al., 2014). His laboratory is now seeking to understand how the cells actually generate those patterns. He presented Figure 4-1 to illustrate the functions of the

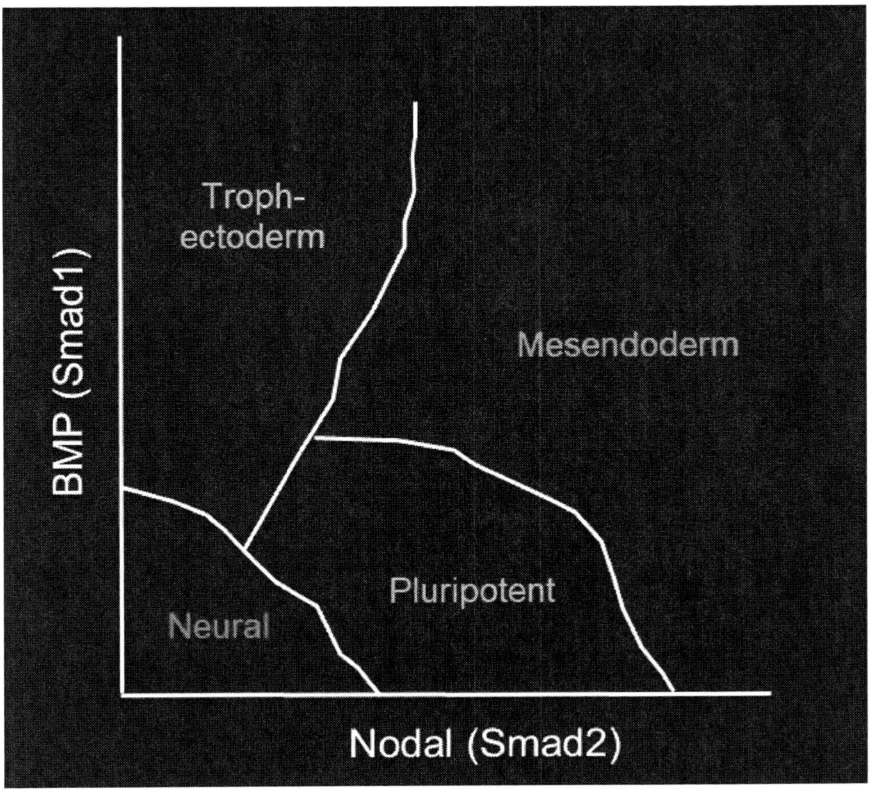

FIGURE 4-1 TGFβ signals (e.g., BMP, Nodal) and cell fates in human embryonic stem cells.
SOURCE: Aryeh Warmflash workshop presentation, January 17, 2020.

signaling pathways that are thought to be involved in differentiating hESCs to each germ layer. BMP (Smad1) is thought to push cells toward the trophectoderm, and some Nodal (Smad2) signaling is required to maintain the pluripotent state. Up-regulating Nodal signaling, together with Wnt, can generate mesoendoderm cells. Down-regulating all of those signals generates neural cells, a subset of the ectodermal germ layer. Warmflash noted that the specific fates within each germ layer can depend on other signals as well. The question is how all of those cell fates are generated along the y-axis (or the BMP signaling) of the diagram in the figure.

Measuring Signaling Dynamics of Key Morphogen Pathways

Warmflash explained how CRISPR-engineered reporters can be used to measure the signaling dynamics of key morphogen pathways, the TGFβ superfamily (BMP and Nodal) and Wnt. It has been established that both Wnt and Nodal signaling are required downstream of BMP4 in order to pattern the gastruloid (Chhabra et al., 2019; Martyn et al., 2018; Warmflash et al., 2014). Time-lapse imaging of hESCs with CRISPR-engineered reporters can be used to create "movies" to watch how these endogenous signals, which are activated downstream of BMP, play out in space and time to generate the patterns observed in hESC colonies. He noted that this technology allows for toggling between sparser culture conditions, in which the cells are mostly responsive to exogenous signals that can be well controlled, and denser micropattern systems, in which the primary controls are endogenous signals.

For the TGFβ superfamily, CRISPR/Cas-tagged alleles were generated for the signal transducer Smad4, which is downstream of both BMP and Activin/Nodal (Heemskerk et al., 2019; Nemashkalo et al., 2017). For the Wnt pathway, β-catenin was tagged to watch Wnt signaling (Massey et al., 2019). Warmflash's team found that BMP signaling is sustained over time (as long as BMP is not inhibited) and that this sustained signaling is necessary for differentiation of cells to CDX2-positive trophectoderm fates (Heemskerk et al., 2019; Nemashkalo et al., 2017). Wnt and Activin/Nodal signaling behave differently than BMP signaling in that they respond adaptively to ligand stimulation, Warmflash said. The Wnt reporter β-catenin starts out at the adherence junctions, and fills the cells when Wnt is added. Then the cells respond adaptively. Despite the constant presence of Wnt in the media, the cells stop Wnt signaling to various degrees; this adaptation is complete at low doses and partial at higher doses (Massey et al., 2019). Activin/Nodal also creates an adaptive signaling response, but with less dependence on the ligand dose—the cells adapt almost completely within about 4 hours, independent of the dose (Heemskerk et al., 2019).

To understand how these patterns are generated, Warmflash and his colleagues looked into the hESC colonies where these signals play out. Warmflash noted that BMP signals are exogenous, but Wnt and Activin/Nodal signals are endogenous. He presented a movie quantifying what happens when a cell colony is treated with BMP4. BMP signaling is initially widespread, but it is then restricted to the colony border where the signaling is sustained (Heemskerk et al., 2019). Initially, the entire colony responds to this high dose of growth factor, but then there is a hollowing out at the center of the colony, with the signal only sustained at the edge, he said. This is consistent with the finding that sustained BMP signaling is needed to generate CDX2-positive trophectoderm. Because BMP signaling is only sustained at the edge of the colony, CDX2-positive trophectoderm can only be generated there. Another movie demonstrated the dynamics of Wnt signaling, which is initially activated close to the edge and spreads inward, with linear propagation of the signal through the colony at a constant rate (Chhabra et al., 2019). In other words, a wave of Wnt signaling moves through the colony from the edge inward. Wnt signaling reaches well beyond the region of mesoderm differentiation, he added. Following the wave of Wnt signaling, Nodal is activated. A wave of Nodal signaling then propagates through the colony and induces mesodermal differentiation in its wake in a certain region of the colony (Heemskerk et al., 2019).

Warmflash summarized this sequence of events in the following way: (1) BMP signaling is initially widespread but then hollows out; (2) a wave of Wnt is triggered through the colony; (3) a wave of Nodal signaling follows the wave of Wnt; and (4) mesoderm differentiation occurs immediately after the wave of Nodal signaling. Both Wnt and Nodal signals reach farther into the colony than primitive streak differentiation, so the signal that controls the positioning of the streak cannot be a simple threshold in either of these pathways. Instead, the cells combinatorially interpret the dynamics of both pathways in making a decision. One hypothesis is that the order in which the cell sees these signals is important, he added. If they see the Wnt signaling and then the Nodal signaling, they will differentiate. If they see the Nodal signaling and then the Wnt signaling, they will not differentiate. This is consistent with data from other laboratories showing directly that the Wnt signal needs to precede the Nodal signal for differentiation.

Molecular Mechanisms That Propagate the Signaling

Warmflash and colleagues have also gained insight into the molecular mechanisms by which these signals propagate. Inhibitor of Wnt Production-2 (IWP2), a small molecule inhibitor of Wnt secretion, is a useful reagent because it inhibits the secretion of Wnt signaling without inhibiting the response to Wnt signaling. Adding IWP2 at different times reveals how the signal propagates through the colony (Chhabra et al., 2019). Unsurprisingly, the earlier that IWP2 is added, the less Wnt signaling is observed. However, they were surprised to find that the Wnt signal travels just as far when the inhibitor is added, even though there is not as much Wnt signaling and new Wnt cannot be produced. This suggests that Wnt is produced near the edge of the colony and then moves inward into the colony via some means of active transport, in a way that is linear in time and does not require production of new Wnt. Therefore, the secretion of new Wnt ligands is dispensable for movement of Wnt signaling, but it increases Wnt levels. Nodal behaves differently when Wnt is inhibited, he said. Wnt is needed to activate the Nodal signaling, but at some point the Nodal signaling becomes self-propagating and independent of upstream pathways, activating itself as it goes through the colony. Nodal has a binary-type phenotype: either it is not activated and stays mostly at the edge, or it is activated everywhere.

Differences Between Micropatterned Cultures and the Embryo

Warmflash observed that the insights they have gained about cell differentiation from dissecting these signals, observing how they regulate each other, and tracking how they propagate through the colony in time would be difficult to obtain using any in vivo system. He provided a brief overview of the differences between the types of micropatterned cultures he described and an actual embryo.

1. In micropatterned cultures the germ "layers" that form are adjacent in the same 2D plane, rather than layered in 3D.
2. The hESC colonies fail to break symmetry: rather than having a primitive streak that forms on the posterior side, as in an embryo, the primitive streak forms as a ring that circles the entire colony.
3. Some extraembryonic lineages are missing in micropatterned cultures: trophectoderm-like cells are present, but not visceral endoderm cells.
4. The glass surface constrains the movements of cells, resulting in a loss of order as cells delaminate.
5. In terms of organismal potential, the system would not develop further if implanted.

Future Directions for Synthetic Embryology

Warmflash emphasized that the goal of this work is not to build embryos from stem cells; rather, the goal is to build systems to answer specific questions about how the embryo works. The current state of knowledge and technical capability warrants simplified systems that can be quantitatively manipulated, measured, and modeled. There is still much to be learned from 2D simplified systems, he said. To learn about later stages or other aspects of development, new systems can then be created that focus on relevant aspects without modeling the entire embryo. For example, patterns can be made at other developmental stages with more complex protocols. This has already been done with the four different states of ectoderm (Britton et al., 2019). Strides have also been made in studying morphogenesis and patterning in 3D, he added. His laboratory has developed controlled ways of taking cells into 3D to model the neural tube. He and his colleagues are also interested in interactions between embryonic and extraembryonic cells. He conceded that it is controversial to put those cell types together, but they are studying the interaction in 2D without developing the cells further. When BMP-differentiated trophectoderm-like cells and ESCs are juxtaposed, the trophectoderm cells induce the gastrulation-like events, including the primitive streak marker Brachyury, in ESCs without the need to add exogenous ligands.

BLASTOIDS: MODELING THE PRE-IMPLANTATION EMBRYO

Nicolas Rivron, a group leader at the Institute of Molecular Biotechnology, Austrian Academy of Sciences, described how his laboratory models early embryonic development in 3D by combining trophoblast stem cells and embryonic stem cells to form blastoids, which model some features of the pre-implantation embryo. He emphasized that the work he would describe is strictly based on mouse stem cells, not human stem cells.

Reciprocity Between Embryo and Placenta

During pregnancy, the placenta is the lifeline that sustains the development of the embryo and the fetus. However, Rivron and colleagues discovered that during the very early developmental stages—before implantation in the uterus—the embryo actually takes care of the future placenta by fueling the proliferation, self-renewal, and morphogenesis of the trophoblast stem cells in the placenta. The embryonic compartment feeds the trophoblast in order to set it apart from the embryo and form the trophectoderm cyst. Through a complex combination of signals, it pushes the trophoblasts to develop and prepares them for implantation inside the uterus. This is interesting from an evolutionary perspective, Rivron remarked, because "at this early stage, the embryo invests in its own future."

Creating a Blastoid

To frame his laboratory's work on blastoids, Rivron presented a movie depicting the very early stages of mammalian development. At day 4.5, the mouse blastocyst comprises about 100 cells and is still floating inside the uterus. At this point it already contains three cell types: the epiblast that will form the full embryo, the primitive endoderm, and the trophectoderm (see Figure 4-2). Although this blastocyst could implant inside the uterus, Rivron and colleagues put it in culture and expand the stem cells that it contains. ESCs are dependent on Wnt and LIF, and trophoblast stem cells (TSCs) are dependent on fibroblast growth factor 4 (FGF4) and TGFβ ligands, Rivron said. Those cells are frozen in time and can be reinjected back into an embryo, where they will contribute to their respective embryonic and placental compartments. In Rivron's laboratory, those cells are recombined in a dish to promote self-organization into a structure that is remarkably similar to the blastocyst. Rivron calls this structure a "blastoid." He underlined two elements that are experimental advantages to blastoids: (1) they can generate large numbers of blastoids because this process does not require embryos every time, and (2) they can genetically edit the stem cells before the blastoid is formed.

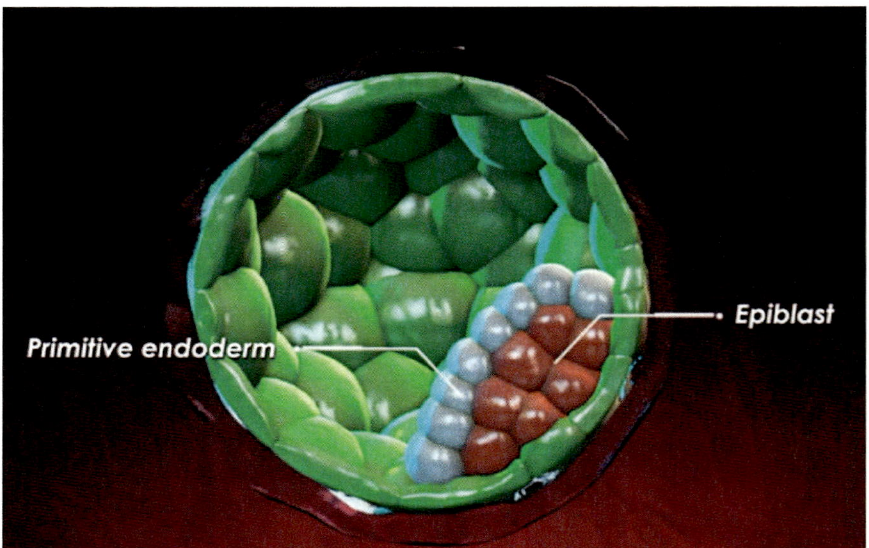

FIGURE 4-2 Mouse blastocyst at day 4.5 (100 cells).
SOURCE: Nicolas Rivron workshop presentation, January 17, 2020.

Rivron noted that since their first publication describing the creation of mouse blastoids in 2018 (Rivron et al., 2018b), three subsequent publications have presented slightly different ways of making mouse blastoids (Kime et al., 2019; Li et al., 2019; Sozen et al., 2019). The approach used by Rivron and colleagues was to first seed ESCs on non-adherent microwells made of a hydrogel (diameter: 200 micrometers). Because the surface is non-adherent, the cells have no other choice but to adhere with each other and aggregate. Once small clusters were formed, they seeded the TSCs on top of them. When they screened for factors that are present during blastocyst formation, they found that the cells remember where they come from and start talking to each other, spontaneously organizing into the structures.

Features of Blastoids

Rivron provided an overview of the features of the blastoid. He explained that the blastoids make analogs of the three cell types that form the blastocyst—epiblast, trophoblast, and primitive endoderm—which later develop into the placenta, yolk sac, and body to form the whole organism. His view is that blastoids do not have organismic potential because development is a historical process that starts with the fertilization of an egg and ends up with the delivery 21 days later (for the mouse). Blastoids are used to model a very short window of time of only 1–3 days. However, the cells at this stage do have the NANOG-positive cells and OCT4-positive cells that will eventually form the body as well as the CDX2-positive cells that will form the placenta. The niche is also permissive for the generation of PDGF-alpha positive cells and GATA6-positive primitive endoderm cells that will form the yolk sac, which is the second extraembryonic tissue.

Blastoids are morphologically similar to blastocysts, Rivron said. They also form very efficiently, with beautiful structures emerging within just 48 hours. In his first series of studies using the microwells containing the appropriate numbers of cells (i.e., 8 ESCs and 20 TSCs), he observed a rate of self-organization to blastoid structure of greater than 70 percent. Subsequently, he has attained levels greater than 90 percent. Rivron added that the yield of blastoids is highly dependent on both the absolute numbers and the ratio of ESCs to TSCs. A comparison of blastoid systems with the actual blastocyst reveals that the blastoid systems have high fidelity and can implant when transferred into the uterus of mice, where the blastoids induce the formation of the uterine cocoon, termed *decidua*. However, the blastoids collapse and cannot develop further after 2 days. In investigating why the blastoids lack the potential for future development, Rivron's group found interesting reactions occurring in the decidua. For example, his group observed the formation of ALDH3A1-positive cells, which has been shown to be specific to the implantation of blastocysts, a marker that suggests a similarity to the implantation process of blastoids. Further characterization revealed CDX2-positive cells, which form the placenta, as well as many other relevant cell types. He concluded that, in the uterus, blastoids can initiate implantation and development in a way that is similar to blastocysts, including the formation of decidua-like structures. However, the cell types in the blastoids were far from properly organized. Box 4-2 is an overview of the blastoid's defining features as presented by Rivron.

The Cooperative Life of Embryo Cells

Rivron's laboratory focuses on understanding the cooperation between cell types in the embryo. More specifically, he and his colleagues look at the autonomous, self-organizing, and cooperative behaviors that lead to the compartmentalization of the conceptus.[4] A flow of information between the future embryo and the extraembryonic tissues facilitates synchronization and establishes developmental checkpoints of development.

Systematic Inventory of Embryonic Inductions

Rivron explained that his group is able to generate trophospheres using the same process for generating blastoids, but without the presence of the embryonic cells. Comparing the blastoids and trophospheres allows for establishing a proxy for the influence of the embryonic cells on the trophoblast cells. He presented single-cell RNA sequencing experiments and a T-distributed stochastic neighbor embedding plot of single blastoid cells, single trophosphere cells, and single TSCs in 2D, which illustrated the

BOX 4-2
Key Features of the Blastoid

- Blastoids model blastocyst development.
- Communication between embryonic stems cells and trophoblast stem cells drives the development of blastoids.
- Blastoids recapitulate aspects of implantation and early development in utero.

SOURCE: Nicolas Rivron workshop presentation, January 17, 2020.

[4]The term *conceptus* was defined in a recent publication as "the products of conception at all stages of development from zygote to birth. These include the embryo proper, the fetus, the placenta, and all extraembryonic membranes" (Hyun et al., 2020, p. 170).

transcriptome shifts occurring upon crosstalk between the trophoblast and embryonic cells. This shift was used, he said, to deeply analyze the effects of the embryonic cells on the trophoblast cells—so-called embryonic inductions. By developing a list of signaling pathways, the group discovered that the embryonic cells strongly influence the development of the trophoblast cells. The embryonic cells produce a range of different factors (e.g., FGF4, Nodal, BMP4, BMP7, and some Wnts) that activate the MAP kinase and TGFβ and Wnt signaling pathways, among others, in the trophoblast.

Further functional analysis of these embryonic inductions demonstrated that embryonic cells regulate trophoblast proliferation and self-renewal, Rivron said. Previous work showed that FGF is inducing the proliferation of the trophoblast cells that are in contact with the embryonic cells and that go on to form the placenta. On the other side of the blastocyst cavity, the cells that are away from the embryonic inductions are differentiating and acquire functions that allow them to mediate implantation inside the uterus. Rivron and colleagues were able to show that the presence of the embryonic cells induces proliferation and self-renewal of the trophoblast in blastoids (Rivron et al., 2018b). By contrast, proliferation was not induced in trophospheres in which those cells were absent. Thus, the blastoids were clearly recapitulating the only known induction, he noted.

In an experiment looking at the TGFβ pathway, Rivron and colleagues compared the diameter of the cystic structures between blastoids and trophospheres (Rivron et al., 2018b). Although trophospheres are smaller than blastoids, they determined that it was possible to apply the factors produced by ESCs (BMP4 and Nodal) on top of the trophospheres. This causes the trophospheres to swell. By counting the number of cells, they determined that Nodal and BMP4 were not inducing proliferation of the cells; rather, they were just inducing the spreading of the structure. Because the researchers were able to perform this analysis on a huge number of blastoids and trophospheres, they were able to identify small effects that would be difficult to pinpoint by analyzing limited numbers of actual blastocysts. Rivron highlighted this as a strong example of an advantage of embryo models. Embryo models can also be used to generate specific knockouts only in one compartment, he added. The trophectoderm stopped swelling when Nodal was specifically knocked out in the embryonic cells, indicating that Nodal is an embryonic inducer that regulates trophectoderm swelling. Furthermore, they discovered that one of the targets of Nodal in the trophoblast, KLF6-positive cells, regulates trophectoderm swelling and likely plays a role in epithelial morphogenetics.

Rivron emphasized that embryonic inductions are important in inducing trophoblast proliferation and self-renewal by (1) maintaining trophectoderm core transcription factors, (2) preventing differentiation, and (3) regulating trophectoderm epithelial morphogenesis. Together, these embryonic inductions also prepare and maintain the potential of trophoblasts to implant inside the uterus. He explained that there is a window of opportunity for trophoblasts to implant and that if the cells differentiate into post-implantation placental cell types, they lose the capacity to implant into the uterus. This is demonstrated in the largely diminished potential to implant observed in trophospheres, which stop proliferating and begin to differentiate in the absence of those embryonic inductions. These findings have implications for addressing the high rate of implantation failure in human pregnancies, he noted. These types of embryo models also hold potential for addressing clinical issues—for example, treating infertility, improving in vitro fertilization, designing new contraceptives, and preventing disease (Hyun et al., 2020; Rivron et al., 2018a).

MICROFLUIDIC STEM CELL MODEL OF PERI-IMPLANTATION

Jianping Fu, an associate professor of biomedical and mechanical engineering and an associate professor of cell and developmental biology at the University of Michigan, discussed stem cell models of peri-implantation human development. His laboratory uses human pluripotent stem cells (hPSCs)—both induced pluripotent stem cells and hESCs—to develop sensitive models for studying pre-implantation human development. He said that investigating many important questions about human development does not require generating complete synthetic structures that include all of the embryonic or extraembryonic images.

Overview of Peri-Implantation Human Embryonic Development

Fu began with an overview of peri-implantation human development. He highlighted the initial notable embryonic events that occur after the blastocyst implants into the maternal uterus. First is the spontaneous formation of the pro-amniotic cavity. The epiblast next to the invading trophoblast then spontaneously differentiates into the amniotic ectoderm, while the remaining epiblast next to the hypoblast may remain pluripotent. Soon after these symmetry-breaking events, the anterior–posterior axis is established, and the posterior end of the epiblast transitions to establish the three different germ layers. After implantation but before gastrulation, another cell type appears—the primordial germ cell, which is a precursor for all of the sex cells that are responsible for human reproduction as well as human evolution.

Self-Organized Development of Stem Cell Models of Peri-Implantation

When the researchers in Fu's laboratory initiated this work, they were not planning to develop systems to model peri-implantation in human development. However, as they developed a 3D culture environment for the control experiment (in which they did not add any exogenous signals to the culture), they observed that hPSCs began to self-organize. The cells developed multicellular structures and underwent morphogenetic events similar to those expected during peri-implantation of human development. First, the hPSCs undergo lumenogenesis to form a cavity. Soon after, the cells begin to change shape, becoming more squamous and flattened, with protrusions beginning to extend from the basal surfaces at the same time (Shao et al., 2017a,b). The researchers determined that the cells were differentiated from hPSCs, and they ultimately characterized these cells as amniotic ectoderm–like cells. The 3D culture environment drove most of the cells to differentiate into uniformly squamous amniotic ectoderm-like cysts, but in about 5–10 percent of the cysts, they observed asymmetry as well as spontaneous symmetry-breaking events. Fu presented an example of this asymmetry. After forming a cavity, some of the cells at one pole of the cyst started to differentiate into squamous amniotic ectoderm–like cells, while the rest of cells remained undifferentiated columnar epiblast-like cells.

Co-staining the cells for pluripotency markers (e.g., NANOG, OCT4, SOX2) suggested that the undifferentiated cells would remain as undifferentiated pluripotent cells, Fu said. When the differentiated cells were stained, only the squamous differentiated cells stained positive for what are thought to be amniotic ectoderm markers. Yet another subpopulation of cells appeared to be mimicking gastrulation-like events that were occurring after lumenogenesis, cavity formation, symmetry breaking, and cell differentiation. These cells, which were disseminating from the undifferentiated epiblast compartment, stained positive for canonical markers associated with gastrulation and began to lose expression for NANOG.

Autonomous BMP Signaling Drives Amniotic Differentiation

Fu and colleagues investigated the molecular mechanisms for driving amniotic cell differentiation from hPSCs in their 3D culture environment. Their model did not have any exogenous external signals driving the stem cells to differentiate, so they looked at BMP signaling pathways. Staining the cells for phosphorylated SMAD, the downstream effector for BMP signaling, suggested that when the cells start to differentiate, they autonomously activate BMP signaling. Blocking BMP signaling enabled the researchers to rescue the pluripotency of the cells in the cadre. Fu said that this observation about autonomous expression or autonomous activation of BMP signaling in amniotic ectoderm–like cells is consistent with available data generated from post-implantation monkey embryos. BMP4 is almost exclusively expressed in the amniotic ectoderm compartment of those monkey embryos, and MSX2—a downstream BMP target gene—is also clearly expressed (Sasaki et al., 2016).

Controlled Microfluidic Modeling of Human Embryo Development

Conventional 3D culture environments can be used to generate self-organizing multicellular structures that bear similarities to certain facets of human development, Fu said. However, these systems offer limited controllability and reproducibility. He illustrated this using data from some of his group's experiments. Although there are clear examples of asymmetric tissue in some cysts, different degrees of progressive development and differentiation are observed in the cysts overall. It is this heterogeneity that limits the conventional 3D culture's controllability and reproducibility and, by extension, limits the utility of these systems for mechanistic investigations.

Over the past several years Fu and colleagues have leveraged their expertise in microengineering and microfluidics to enhance controllability through controlled microfluidic modeling of human embryo development (Zheng et al., 2019). This system features a simple microfluidic structure, he explained. The microfluidic device contains an induction channel and a cell-loading channel; gels are loaded into the central channel between the other two. During gelation, the gel contracts due to surface tension, causing the gel to autonomously generate gel pockets that form between the supporting posts. hPSCs are loaded into the cell-loading channel and the device is tilted 90 degrees for 10 minutes. Many of the cells spontaneously settle into each of the gel pockets; later, the floating cells can gently be removed. In this way microfluidics makes it possible to create assays that offer superior controllability, reproducibility, and scalability.

Fu described the first set of experiments he and his colleagues performed with the microfluidic modeling system. No exogenous inductive signals were added to jog the stem cells to differentiate, so all the cells would remain pluripotent, he noted. As soon as the hPSCs started touching each other, they began to coalesce into a community and spontaneously underwent lumenogenesis, forming cavities of epiblast-like cysts in a synchronized way.[5] He said that this type of microfluidic system is scalable and compatible with live imaging, enabling investigation of the cells' signaling

[5]Fu noted that this is an established lumenogenic property of hPSCs.

dynamics, signaling propagation, and the inductive signals that drive the formation of different compartments.

Asymmetric BMP Stimulation Induces Embryonic-Like Sac Formation

In the second set of experiments, Fu and colleagues decided to add BMP4 into one of the top channels (Zheng et al., 2019). They had established in their previous studies that BMP4 signaling is sufficient to drive hPSCs to differentiate into amniotic ectoderm–like cells. In the bottom cell-loading channel, there were no exogenous inductive signals. When the cells underwent lumenogenesis, the cells directly exposed to BMP4 stimulation spontaneously differentiated into amniotic ectoderm–like cells. However, because only a portion of the cells in each cell colony were directly exposed to BMP4, they form asymmetrical bipolar embryonic-like structure. Once the top portion of cells differentiated into amniotic ectoderm–like cells, these amniotic cells began secreting inductive signals to drive the continuous development of the bottom portion of undifferentiated cells to spontaneously undergo gastrulation-like events. At certain time points, molecular asymmetry was very evident in the stem cells: only the cells that were directly exposed to BMP4 stimulation expressed TFAP2A, the gastrulating cells expressed T/Brachyury and were continuously differentiating, and all of the cells expressed CDX2. (CDX2 is an extraembryonic marker, but it also expresses in the posterior primitive streak.) Fu showed a video demonstrating this patterning. The cells formed a cavity and the top cells exposed to BMP4 became increasingly squamous and flattened. Soon after, the cells started to disseminate from the opposite pole. Fu said that he and his colleagues cease all experiments at day 3 or 4 because after that point the entire structure will disassemble and collapse, with gastrulating cells disseminating in an uncontrollable fashion.

Emergence of Primordial Germ Cell–Like Cells in Embryonic-Like Sac

Fu's laboratory has also used the microfluidic model system to look at primordial germ cells, the important cell lineage developed in embryonic tissue that appears post-implantation but before gastrulation (Kobayashi et al., 2017; Sasaki et al., 2016). In that case cells were stained with canonical markers SOX17, NANOG, and TFAP2C, and the triple-positive cells were identified as primordial germ cell–like cells, which began to appear at early time points in a scattered fashion. Soon after, these cells began to accumulate toward the junction between the amniotic ectoderm compartment and the gastrulating epiblast-like cell compartment. The researchers also observed some interesting cell dynamics, suggesting that this type of system would be informative for examining the origin and lineage development of primordial germ cells in early human embryonic development.

Comparative Transcriptome Analysis with Primate Monkey Embryo Data

As an in vitro system, the system developed by Fu's laboratory is compatible with the use of downstream genomic analysis and single-cell transcriptome profiling to identify cell types and lineage markers. The researchers have also used comparative transcriptome analysis to compare the cell types generated by their synthetic system with cell types developed from primate monkey embryos (Nakamura et al., 2016). According to Fu, the gastrulating cells generated by their system are similar to the gastrulating cells from the monkey embryos. The researchers also compared the primordial germ cell–like cells generated by the system with those generated in monkey and human embryos and other in vitro culture models (Kobayashi et al., 2017; Kojima et al., 2017; Sasaki et al., 2016). The primordial–germ cell–like cells generated by the microfluidic system compared well with those generated in other in vitro culture models, Fu said.

PANEL DISCUSSION

Toward More Unified Terminology

Given the range of the terminology being used in these models (e.g., blastoids, gastruloids, neuruloids, synthetic embryos, embryoids), Clark suggested trying to unify the terms that scientists use to discuss this work—and to do it in a way that does not cause alarm among the general public. Warmflash described "synthetic embryo" as an inappropriate term, for instance; embryo should not be part of the name because these models do not have organismal potential. He suggested promoting uniform use of the "-oid" suffix to indicate that something is an in vitro model that aims to capture features of a stage of development (e.g., a blastoid is an in vitro model intended to capture something about the blastocyst stage, but it is not a real blastocyst). Rivron agreed that names should be based on what the system is presumed to be modeling, with the "-oid" suffix used to clarify that it is only a model. However, a challenge is that at the outset, the window of development to which the cells are equivalent is unknown. Fu suggested using "stem cell–based models of human development" if a single umbrella term including all of the models is needed.

Molecular-Controlling Influences of Size

A workshop participant asked Brivanlou about the influence of the diameter change on the RNA-sequencing profiles. A major consideration in biology in general and in embryology in particular is the molecular-controlling influences of size: everything has a given thickness and diameter that sometimes changes over time, Brivanlou said. When the size of the cell colonies is shrunk, the center fate is always lost (i.e., ectoderm is lost when the size shifts from 1,000 to 500 microns; mesoderm is lost and only trophectoderm remains when the size shifts from 500 to 125 microns). Further work in Brivanlou's laboratory has shown that the cells have a "magic ruler" that measures the distance from the edge, indicating that the patterns are controlled from the edge, not from the center. The researchers in Brivanlou's lab have defined two features of that ruler: (1) physical edge sensing that is dictated and imposed by the BMP receptor and (2) a reaction diffusion whereby BMP4 induces the direct expression of its own inhibitor, NOGIN. In no other species, including nonhuman primates, is BMP4 able to directly induce the expression of its own inhibitor. This creates a Turing pattern, in which NOGIN diffuses much faster from the edge toward the center and completely blocks the effect of BMP4 coming from trophectoderm.

Using Blastoids to Model Developmental Potential

Rivron was asked if he had tried adding primitive endoderm lineage to the blastoid model in order to look at the effect on implantation developmental potential. His team did so in the original protocol, he answered, and primitive endoderm did form, but the numbers were not sufficient. His team's approach is to push ESCs to form primitive endoderm cells by exposing cells to certain factors using specific "cocktails" that can efficiently form primitive endoderm cells. Next, they developed an assay to functionally test whether more primitive endoderm cells would help to support further development. They observed a higher propensity for the egg cylinder to develop after the induction of primitive endoderm cells, suggesting that the epiblast may develop in synergy with the primitive endoderm. Primitive endoderm may be one of many elements required for blastoids to take the next developmental step, Rivron surmised. He noted that this type of work demonstrates certain advantages of using stem cell–based embryo models over the classical approach to embryology, which involves knocking out genes in actual embryos and looking for a phenotype. This approach is limited to genes that provide a good phenotype and can actually be studied using the genetic knockout; those genes have now been largely exhausted. Embryo models offer a new approach that works in the opposite direction:

starting with a minimal structure (i.e., rudimentary blastoid) and building it up with increasing complexity to see if it progresses through the developmental steps. This bottom-up approach to embryology allows for identifying minimal features that are necessary for development but could not be seen before.

Stable Endpoints Versus Continuous Differentiation in Model Systems

A workshop participant asked whether stem cell–based systems end at defined states or have continuous differentiation and developmental processes, which has implications for the propagation and development of different cell types. Warmflash said that the systems he uses will continue to develop, but their fidelity diminishes over time because the systems have been engineered to model a specific stage. The cell types will mature because they are programmed to keep developing, but they will lose organization due to the limitations of 2D culture systems. In his work on frog development, Brivanlou observed a linear progression over time in transitions of cell fates. The germ layers were produced, and then posterior patterning kicked in within the germ layers; morphogenesis added another layer of complexity. Cell fates continue to change as a function of time—frogs can develop from a single cell to 40 million cells in only 48 hours. In addition to this transition of cell states, other issues in embryology include the ability of a cell to acquire a fate or to undergo a transition in time and space. In contrast to the natural environment, in which a developing system progresses without extrinsic information, experimental conditions involve adding extrinsic information (e.g., BMP4, Wnt, and/or Nodal) and then measuring what the cells can do in that specific milieu within a very small window of transition time.

Human Versus Nonhuman Model Systems

Speakers were asked whether the models that had been discussed might eventually obviate the need to study human embryonic material directly. A workshop participant went on to ask which elements might be essential to continue studying using human material versus those that might be replaced with models in nonhuman primates or other species. Brivanlou replied that limits on the length of modeling notwithstanding, there will never be enough biological material—from humans, nonhuman primates, or other species—available to perform quantitative measurements with the level of resolution offered by synthetic model systems.

Validating Human-Specific Features of Synthetic Models

Kriegstein asked the panelists to consider how it will be possible to validate the human-specific features of these models without the use of animal models and given the limited access to human tissue. RNA-sequencing approaches can be used, Brivanlou answered. For example, his laboratory has used this approach to provide direct evidence that a splice isoform of the Huntington gene only exists in hominids. More difficult to test are, for example, species-specific signaling interactions and reaction diffusions. However, Brivanlou predicted that some of the models described by the panelists would ultimately allow for that type of testing. CRISPR/Cas9 can already be used to perform tracing at resolutions never achieved before, he added. He expressed hope that quantitative tools would be developed to demonstrate the speed of NOGIN with BMP4 in real time in a human model.

Huntington's Disease Phenotype in the Gastrula Stage

Kriegstein remarked that Huntington's disease tends to manifest several decades after birth, so the gastrula-stage phenotype identified by Brivanlou seems to appear earlier than expected. Brivanlou replied that this was also a surprise to him. Huntington's disease is caused by an insertion of CAG-repeats in a gene called *Huntingtin* (*HTT*). Different individuals have CAG-repeats of different lengths in their *HTT* gene, and the onset of the disease is CAG-length-dependent, with longer insertions corresponding to an earlier manifestation of the disease. The earliest recorded death from Huntington's disease is 18 months of age, Brivanlou said. Comparative studies in a variety of species suggest that a maternal rescue component kicks in and mediates many of the early effects of the mutation, which may account for why the disease tends to manifest later in life. The loss of both *Huntingtin* alleles ($HTT^{-/-}$) leads to embryonic lethality, demonstrating that the gene is necessary for gastrulation and that it has independent functions beyond the nervous system. The gene is expressed in the fertilized egg and then expressed ubiquitously in all adult cell types. If the mutation were a dominant mutation, it follows that the earliest effect of the mutant would occur at the earliest time point of biological activity, Brivanlou said. Furthermore, a mouse model study found that if a pulse of Huntington mutant is given to an early embryo and then the activity is retracted, the adult will manifest Huntington's disease symptoms, he noted.

Markers of Peri-Implantation Development

Fu was asked how he determines that he is not actually studying trophoblast differentiation instead of peri-implantation development. A key diagnostic marker to identify developmental stage is the appearance of primordial germ cell–like stem cells in the amniotic ectoderm compartment, Fu said, because primordial germ cells only appear post-implantation and before gastrulation. This suggests that the amniotic ectoderm compartment corresponds to the amniotic compartment in the peri-implantation human embryo. However, the underlying question of whether his lab has established the equivalency of the cell types generated in their in vitro models cannot be answered until data become available that allow them to perform comparisons with in vivo human or primate embryos.

Precursor of Germ Cells

Martin Pera asked Fu if lineage tracing had been used to look for the precursor of the germ cells. Fu replied that he has a grant pending with the aim of answering that specific question. He added that these synthetic models provide powerful experimental platforms for advancing fundamental understanding about human development, particularly for discovering essential features of developmental mechanisms at a detailed molecular level.

5

Comparative Embryonic Development Across Species

Important Points Highlighted by Individual Speakers

- Aneuploidy is a leading cause of human embryo loss and in vitro fertilization failure. Rhesus macaque pre-implantation embryos are useful models to study because they have incidences of micronucleation, aneuploidy, and cellular fragmentation that are nearly equal to those in human embryos. Equine and bovine embryos share some of these features at a similar frequency, but mouse embryos exhibit far lower levels of these characteristics. (Chavez)
- Models for aneuploidy related to maternal age are needed because the primates being studied are often relatively young. Mouse models could be useful for learning about maternal age-related aneuploidy and post-implantation, while the monkey would be useful for studying pre-implantation development. (Chavez)
- Although further work is warranted, nonhuman primate pluripotent cells are not equivalent to human cells for modeling trophoblast differentiation. However, rhesus macaque embryos and trophoblast stem cells may offer enhanced translatability for modeling human embryos. (Golos)

- Cells derived from the neural crest are believed to be involved in many pathologies, including birth defects such as orofacial clefts and cancers. The specification of neural crest cells happens earlier than originally thought, in a region of the pre-gastrula epiblast. (García-Castro)
- It is possible to rapidly derive neural crest cells from human embryonic stem cells cultured in defined media and treated with Wnt, an approach that circumvents some of the challenges with accessing human embryos to study. (García-Castro)
- Expanded-potential stem cells generated either from the embryo or from somatic cells can self-organize and generate a blastocyst-like structure that can model some events in the post-implantation period. Expanded-potential stem cells can be cultured to give rise to functional trophoblast, embryonic, and primitive endoderm stem cell lines. (Wu)

The fourth session of the workshop focused on comparative embryonic development across species. The session's objectives were to understand the similarities and differences between nonhuman embryos, embryo models (e.g., chimeras), and human embryos and to identify scientific questions that may necessitate the study of human embryos. The session was moderated by Jianping Fu.

CROSS-SPECIES COMPARISON OF PRE-IMPLANTATION CHROMOSOMAL INSTABILITY

Shawn Chavez, an assistant professor in the Division of Reproductive and Developmental Sciences at Oregon Health & Science University, provided a comparison of pre-implantation chromosomal instability among different mammalian species, focusing on the prevalence of aneuploidy in pre-implantation embryos and mechanisms of mitotic mis-segregation and chromosome sequestering by micronuclei.

Aneuploidy in Pre-Implantation Embryos

Although in vitro fertilization (IVF) use has continued to increase each year, Chavez said, the success of IVF as measured by live births has not increased beyond 30–35 percent for decades. A leading cause of IVF failure and embryo loss is the presence of aneuploidy, which affects about

50–80 percent of cleavage-stage human embryos (Chavez et al., 2012; Chow et al., 2014; Huang et al., 2015; Johnson et al., 2010; McCoy, 2015; Vanneste et al., 2009a,b). Although an estimated 50 percent or more aneuploid embryos will arrest, they can still form blastocysts and may be morphologically indistinguishable from chromosomally normal (i.e., euploid) embryos. Both meiotic and mitotic errors contribute to aneuploidy, she noted. Until recently, errors involving chromosomal mis-segregation in oocytes during meiosis were considered the primary reason for aneuploidy, especially in cases of advanced maternal age. In maternal age-related aneuploidy, oocytes contribute approximately 90 percent of the meiotic errors. However, errors involving chromosomal mis-segregation during mitosis occur with equal frequency or perhaps even greater frequency than meiotic errors, irrespective of maternal age or fertility status.

Aneuploidies are diagnosed using pre-implantation genetic testing for aneuploidy (PGT-A), formerly known as pre-implantation genetic screening, Chavez said. PGT-A is associated with various risks and disadvantages based on the stage of development at which the biopsy occurs: polar body biopsy of a zygote, blastomere biopsy during cleavage stage, or trophectoderm biopsy of a blastocyst. At the zygote stage, PGT-A only detects meiotic errors. The biopsy of blastomeres at the cleavage-stage suffers from a high incidence of mosaicism,[1] and there is evidence that the blastocyst stage is similarly mosaic. Biopsy performed during the blastocyst stage may also require extended culture. Regardless of the stage, all biopsies are considered invasive and may be detrimental to embryonic development.

Aneuploidy Frequency in Early Cleavage-Stage Embryos Across Mammals

Chavez outlined what is known about the range of aneuploidy frequency at the early cleavage stage across different mammalian species. As previously stated, aneuploidy occurs in about 50–80 percent of human embryos and in around 74 percent of nonhuman primates, specifically rhesus macaque embryos (Daughtry et al., 2019). In the cow, aneuploidy rates range from 32 to 85 percent in early cleavage-stage embryos (Destouni et al., 2016; Hornak et al., 2016; Tšuiko et al., 2017). This is a large range, Chavez said, but the majority of the studies were done using in vitro matured eggs, and in vitro maturation is known to increase aneuploidy due to both meiotic and mitotic errors. In the horse, the aneuploidy frequency is not yet known, although studies are ongoing using in vitro matured eggs. In a natural setting (i.e., no chemical induction), the mouse exhibits the least

[1]Mosaicism is the presence of more than one karyotypically distinct cell lineage in a single embryo (McCoy, 2017).

amount of aneuploidy (1 to 4 percent) (Bolton et al., 2016; Lightfoot et al., 2006; Macaulay et al., 2015; Treff et al., 2016), but this increases with maternal age and in vitro maturation.

Research Questions Regarding Aneuploidy in Pre-Implantation Embryos

Further research on aneuploidy in pre-implantation embryos is needed, Chavez said. One area to explore is the underlying mechanisms that may help explain why there is such a high incidence of aneuploidy in pre-implantation embryos. Another question to investigate is whether live cell imaging—with or without labeled markers—can be used to dissect those mechanisms and to assess embryo developmental potential. Her laboratory focuses on the nuclear structure where the DNA is located, but she is also looking at cytoskeletal structure, given the cross-communication between those components. Determining whether there are corrective natural or therapeutic means to overcome chromosomal instability and aneuploidy generated during pre-implantation development should also be explored, Chavez said, adding that this area of research on pre-implantation development has the greatest potential to help the IVF community.

Mechanisms of Mitotic Mis-Segregation and Sequestering by Micronuclei

Current knowledge about four mechanisms of aneuploidy has been derived primarily from cancer cells and, more recently, from mouse embryos, Chavez said. Abnormal centrosome numbers—either too few or too many centrosomes—can have consequences such as multipolar divisions. Defective spindle attachments involve some kind of non-attachment or abnormal attachment. Compromised cell cycle checkpoints suggest that abnormal events such as an anaphase lagging chromosome go unrecognized and that the embryo divides before it has a chance to line up on the spindle; this is an area in which much of the mouse embryo work has been done. Loss of or prolonged chromosome adhesion are mechanisms by which chromosomes come apart too soon or stick together too much.

Regardless of the mechanism of aneuploidy, Chavez said, the embryo knows that a chromosome has been mis-segregated. This has been demonstrated by staining cleavage-stage embryos with DAPI for DNA as well as by using the nuclear envelope marker LMNB1 to show that mis-segregated chromosomes have been encapsulated in micronuclei during the next mitotic division (Chavez et al., 2012). These micronuclei have also been observed in nonhuman primates (Daughtry et al., 2019), the horse (Brooks et al., 2019), and the cow; however, micronuclei formation is rarely observed in the early cleavage stages of the mouse (Chavez et al., 2014). Knowledge about the potential fate of these chromosome-containing micronuclei has been gleaned from cancer cells as well as from bovine and mouse embryos (Brooks et al., 2019; Chavez et al., 2012; Crasta et al., 2012; Daughtry et al., 2019; Liu et al., 2018; Vazquez-Diez et al., 2016; Zhang et al., 2015). One fate is unilateral inheritance, whereby the micronucleus that has formed goes on to replicate and divide just like the primary nucleus, so it is propagated with development. This has been demonstrated in bovine embryos at the early cleavage stage, in mouse embryos at the morula stage, and in cancer cells. Another fate is nuclear fusion, in which the nuclear envelope breaks down and the micronucleus fuses back with the primary nucleus. Work on cancer cells indicates that this is highly detrimental, because these micronuclei have undergone severe mutations and chromosome chaos.

Aneuploidy and Chromosome Loss Due to Cellular Fragmentation

Research on human and rhesus embryos has shown that one phenotype highly associated with micronuclei formation is a process called cellular fragmentation, Chavez said. DAPI, LMNBI, and CENP-A staining techniques have been used to show that a highly fragmented embryo can contain DNA not just in micronuclei, but also within cellular fragments. In fact, aneuploidy is often, but not always, associated with cellular fragmentation (Alikani et al., 1999; Antczak and Van Blerkom, 1999; Buster et al., 1985; Chavez et al., 2012; Dozortsev et al., 1998; Hardy et al., 2001; Pereda and Croxatto, 1978; Rambags et al., 2005). This process is observed in about 50 percent or more primate and equine embryos and about 15–20 percent of bovine embryos, although it is rarely seen in mouse embryos unless induced experimentally. Cellular fragmentation is distinct from the DNA fragmentation that can occur following cell death late in pre-implantation development and evidence suggests that it occurs in vivo for multiple species, including humans. Fragmented embryos often exhibit chromosome loss from blastomeres, Chavez said, which complicates aneuploidy assessment.

Chavez highlighted a study that she and her colleagues conducted of aneuploidy and chromosome loss via cellular fragmentation in rhesus embryos using single-cell, next-generation sequencing of 254 blastomeres, 42 polar bodies, and 175 cellular fragments isolated from 50 cleavage-stage embryos (Daughtry et al., 2019). The majority of the polar bodies, whose identity was confirmed by single-nucleotide polymorphism genotyping, were chromosomally normal. However, only about one-quarter of the blastomeres were completely normal; high degrees of aneuploidy and mosaicism were observed in the blastomeres. The researchers also found that the missing chromosomes that had been lost from blastomeres were encapsulated within cellular fragments. There did not appear to be any preferential sequestering of specific chromosomes, and the pieces of chromosomes observed were quite large (6–85 megabases). Multipolar divisions were the most frequent phenotype that resulted in the formation of chromosome-containing cellular fragments, and all of the associated blastomeres exhibited chaotic aneuploidy. However, because not every single embryo exhibited this phenotype, Chavez's group is investigating other mechanisms, such as chromatin or anaphase bridging.

DNA Damage in Chromosome-Containing Cellular Fragments and Micronuclei

Eighteen percent of the rhesus embryos in the study had chromosome-containing fragments, Chavez said, but only 6 percent of all the fragments had DNA detectable by sequencing. Daughtry et al. (2019) surmised that once the cellular fragments encapsulate the DNA, they become highly damaged because they no longer contain a nuclear envelope. Micronuclei can form as early as the zygote stage, but they can also be retained in the blastocyst stage—either as previous or new events—and may have substantial DNA damage. Ongoing work has shown that there are micronuclei in the trophectoderm as well as in the inner cell mass (ICM) of blastocysts; Chavez's team is currently analyzing blastocysts at the single-cell level for aneuploidy and to establish whether DNA damage has occurred. Fluorescent live-cell imaging is being used to identify in real time which cleavage-stage embryos have cellular fragments that contain DNA so that they can be isolated before they start to degrade. The aim is to identify which blastomeres contain DNA so that they can be carried forward for sequencing. The fluorescent labels do not interfere with DNA sequencing, Chavez said.

Chromosomally Mosaic Embryos Can Lead to the Birth of Healthy Offspring

Several years ago, Chavez said, the IVF community was rocked by the finding that in about 50 percent of cases, chromosomally mosaic embryos can result in the live birth of healthy offspring (Greco et al., 2015). Some of these studies have since explored a potential post-implantation mechanism for this phenomenon (Bolton et al., 2016; Fragouli et al., 2017; Gleicher et al., 2016). However, to help the IVF community specifically will require a better understanding of the mechanisms that occur during preimplantation. To explore whether there are selective growth advantages for euploid cells or mechanisms for the elimination of aneuploid cells during pre-implantation development, Chavez and colleagues cultured 92 rhesus embryos with time-lapse imaging, with a blastocyst formation rate of 54.3 percent. At the cleavage stage, 26.5 percent of the embryos were euploid and 32.6 percent were mosaic, suggesting that some of those blastocysts would be chromosomally abnormal to a certain degree.

By returning to the time-lapse imaging, they found that some of these rhesus embryos exhibited cellular fragmentation that was excluded from the rest of the embryo and appeared not to participate in embryo development. About 16 percent of the rhesus blastocysts exhibited blastomere exclusion—that is, upon blastocyst transition one or more of the embryos' blastomeres fails to divide from the 2- to 4-cell stage and is sequestered to the blastocoel. DAPI staining was used to reveal the exclusion of DNA-containing cellular fragments upon embryo hatching. The researchers also found that excluded blastomeres were multi-nucleated, had substantial DNA damage, and were highly chromosomally abnormal. This suggests that blastomere exclusion is at least one of the mechanisms that serves to overcome aneuploidy during pre-implantation development, Chavez said. This mechanism also appears to be conserved across species, because it has also been observed in horse and cow embryos.

In closing, Chavez reiterated that rhesus pre-implantation embryos have the same incidence of micronucleation, aneuploidy, and cellular fragmentation as human embryos. However, models for aneuploidy related to maternal age are still needed, she said, because the monkeys used are relatively young. The mouse model could still be useful for maternal age-related aneuploidy and post-implantation, she said, while the monkey would be useful for modeling pre-implantation development.

TROPHOBLAST DIFFERENTIATION FROM PRIMATE PLURIPOTENT CELLS

Ted Golos, a professor and the chair of the Department of Comparative Biosciences at the University of Wisconsin, considered whether trophoblast differentiation can occur with primate pluripotent cells. He described the formation of embryoid bodies from human embryonic stem cells and the use of rhesus embryoid bodies to model trophoblast differentiation. He also examined the predictive capacity of nonhuman primate embryo model systems.

Breakthroughs in Modeling Trophoblast Differentiation with hESCs

In the mid-1990s, Golos said, James Thomson at the Wisconsin National Primate Research Center modified methods previously used with mouse embryonic stem cells to produce multiple embryonic stem cell (ESC) lines using blastocysts from the rhesus monkey produced in vivo (Thomson et al., 1995). It was also observed that ESCs from the rhesus monkey and the common marmoset can spontaneously give rise to gene expression associated with trophoblasts, because those spontaneously differentiating ESCs initiate the expression of chorionic gonadotropin (CG) and its alpha and beta subunits. Thomson was later able to derive human ESCs (hESCs) based on the spontaneous differentiation and secretion of CG (Thomson et al., 1998). This established that trophoblast formation is also a hallmark of hESCs, which is not, Golos noted, the case for mouse ESC models. This work gave rise to the question of whether primate and human ESCs can provide a system for modeling trophoblast differentiation and placental morphogenesis. Spontaneous differentiation of hESCs to the trophoblast lineage in vitro or in teratomas is of low efficiency; a breakthrough occurred when Xu and colleagues discovered that bone morphogenetic protein 4 (BMP4) or other related ligands can be used to produce a morphologically homogeneous population of cells (Xu et al., 2002). Although it may not have been a homogeneous trophoblast population, this new model clearly had great potential.

Embryoid Body Formation from hESCs

While this work was ongoing with BMP and other ligands, Golos and colleagues decided to use the embryoid body (EB) as an approximation of a spherical embryoid structure, by lifting the hESC colonies and maintaining them in suspension in two-dimensional (2D) culture (Gerami-Naini et al., 2004). They also developed a method for three-dimensional (3D) culture of EBs from hESCs in extracellular matrix by physically inserting EBs into droplets of Matrigel and maintaining them in suspension. Golos explained that EBs in suspension culture initiate the secretion of the "holy trinity" of protein and steroid hormones characteristic of primate placental function: CG, progesterone, and estrogen (the latter is secreted if given an androgenic precursor; see Gerami-Naini et al., 2004). Furthermore, EBs growing in a 3D Matrigel scaffold initiate the sustained secretion of CG as well as of progesterone and estradiol. This established that both 2D and 3D Matrigel environments were able to support placenta trophoblast secretions.

Adaptation of hESC Paradigms to In Vivo Implantation

Next, Golos and colleagues sought to adapt these paradigms to a system that might eventually mimic implantation. Although they had seen outgrowths into Matrigel in the previous work with embryoid bodies, they had not seen villous morphogenesis. Because the morphogenesis of chorionic villi and implantation are similar—but not identical—between humans and macaques, they used rhesus ESCs for the BMP4 differentiation paradigm. They also plated EBs on 2D Matrigel and inserted EBs into a 3D Matrigel environment. However, neither BMP4 nor the 2D/3D Matrigel culture stimulated the secretion of monkey CG or progesterone, nor did they observe any expression of endocrine function when using hormone secretion as the readout for whether mESCs were equivalent to hESCs. To explore whether a non-endocrine differentiation marker would be more productive, they used flow cytometry for the rhesus monkey homolog of HLA-G (i.e., Mamu-AG). In the primary trophoblast cultures, there was clear expression of placenta-specific Mamu-AG with differentiation in the 2D EB culture paradigm.[2] However, one of the rhesus ESC lines did occasionally have outgrowths in which some of the cells expressed Mamu-AG, so the approach was not fully consistent. Coupled with the lack of endocrine differentiation, this called into question the use of CG as a readout and suggested that perhaps the macaque placental endocrine profile may not be appropriate for these approaches.

Use of Rhesus Embryoid Bodies to Model Trophoblast Differentiation

It was established in 1974 that CG is rapidly secreted 10–11 days after implantation in rhesus monkeys. Although CG is somewhat truncated, it is clearly a marker and a signaling mechanism for corpus luteum rescue (Hodgen et al., 1974). Therefore, Golos and colleagues returned to the use of embryos produced in vitro and inserted hatched blastocysts into the 3D Matrigel environment that they had used with EBs (Chang et al., 2018). They observed outgrowths from those blastocysts into the Matrigel as well as the initiation of the secretion of CG, progesterone, and estradiol. This work also provided a good visual depiction of the embryonic structure in the Matrigel. Wispy areas can be observed where the trophoblasts are growing out into the Matrigel as well as digestion degradation of the Matrigel environment, which is consistent with the metalloproteinase expression and secretion that is also seen with the interstitial migration of extravillous trophoblast (EVT) into the maternal decidua. This work suggests that the actual rhesus embryo might be a more appropriate model of trophoblast differentiation than pluripotent cells, Golos said. Recently, Okae et al. (2018) have reported the derivation of human trophoblast stem cells (TSCs). Using the Okae approach, Golos and his colleagues have generated eight macaque (rhesus and cynomolgus) TSC lines and, under the appropriate paradigms, they have been able to use TSC differentiated to syncytiotrophoblast (STB) to initiate substantial monkey CG secretion into the culture medium.

---

[2]Mark Garthwaite and Svetlana Dambaeva, unpublished data.

Predictive Capacity of Nonhuman Primate Embryo Model Systems

To the question of whether nonhuman primate embryo model systems can predict the function of systems made with human cells, Golos said that currently rhesus pluripotent cells are not transparently equivalent to human cells for trophoblast differentiation. In addition to the approaches that Golos described, there are other potential avenues for discovering the differences between rhesus and human pluripotent cells, including differentiation paradigms, receptor complement, feeder cells, trophoblast differentiation niche, maternal factors, genetic background, and organoid aggregates with placental stroma. On the other hand, it is well established that rhesus IVF blastocysts implant in vitro, secrete stereotypical placental hormones, and have invasive trophoblasts that invade and degrade a Matrigel environment. Thus, rhesus embryos might be a tractable system with which to study some of these important processes in early pregnancy. Furthermore, given the limited availability of monkey embryos, rhesus TSCs also could be a high-throughput model for the differentiation of in situ trophoblasts and putative EVT. In addition to forming monkey CG–secreting multinuclear STB and putative EVT, rhesus TSCs express placenta-specific major histocompatibility complex class I molecules; RNA sequencing shows that they appear to be authentic trophoblasts.

Answering Scientific Questions by Studying the Human Embryo

There are a number of scientific questions that could be answered by studying the human embryo, Golos said. Within a few weeks of fertilization, the human embryo has invasive primitive STB that becomes buried in the decidua (West et al., 2019). That invasion process may not be easy to model in nonhuman primates and may require human systems, he said; however, useful information about the peri-implantation period may potentially be gathered from other species. A strength of the nonhuman primate model, he said, is that it provides opportunities to interrogate through pre-implantation embryo manipulation different types of embryonic events that are critical for in vivo placentation, such as villous morphogenesis, spiral artery endovascular migration of EVT, and vessel remodeling. These are experiments that cannot be conducted at the requisite stage of human pregnancy, so toggling back and forth between different kinds of models may be needed in order to answer precise questions about the components that underlie pregnancy success and adverse pregnancy outcomes.

EARLY NEURAL CREST FORMATION: FROM BIRDS TO HUMANS

Martín García-Castro, an associate professor of biomedical sciences at the University of California, Riverside, made a case for pursuing early studies of neural crest cells, both in human and in alternative model organisms. He explained the ontogeny and differentiation potential of the neural crest and described how human neural crest formation can be modeled using pluripotent stem cells.

Neural Crest and Neural Crest Derivatives

In 1868 Wilhelm His used the chicken embryo to pinpoint the cells between the prospective epidermis and the neural ectoderm, which he predicted would also be found at different stages in the elevated neural folds, inside the neural tube, outside the neural tube, and migrating to colonize cranial ganglia (His, 1868). His initially referred to these cells as the intermediate cord, but they were later renamed the neural crest (Marshall, 1879). Subsequent work has shown that these cells arise along the anterior–posterior axis of the embryo at the edge of the neural plate and are marked by the transcription factors Pax7/Pax3 among others. After these cells reach the neural folds, they undergo an epithelial-to-mesenchymal transition to delaminate from the neural tube and migrate extensively through stereotypic pathways in very precise routes, generating a series of neural crest derivatives. Throughout the body, they contribute to neurons and glia of the peripheral nervous system and generate the melanocytes in the skin that provide color and protect from ultraviolet rays. They also make specific derivatives in distinct territories, including cartilage, bone, and connective tissue in the cranial region and sympathoadrenal cells in the trunk. Neural crest derivatives are thought to be involved in one-third of all birth defects, including orofacial clefts and rare syndromes. They also contribute to cancers, including melanoma. Because neural crest cells are involved in so many pathologies, García-Castro said, these cells hold great promise for clinical studies.

Differentiation Potential of Neural Crest

García-Castro described his work, which focuses on the origin of the neural crest and, specifically, trying to understand how it is possible to generate so many different cell types (e.g., neurons, glia, melanocytes, adipocytes, odontoblasts, osteoblasts, chondroblasts, myocytes, oxygen-sensing cells of the carotid body, and thymus mesenchyme) given the putative origin of these cells. The standard story is that after fertilization, cells differentiate to generate epiblast cells, which in turn undergo gastrulation that generates the three germ layers: the endoderm that makes the internal organs; the mesoderm that forms bone, cartilage, adipose tissue, and blood-forming cells; and the ectoderm that produces the central nervous system and the epidermis. Neural crest cells are purportedly derived from the ectoderm and, as such, they are progenitors of the neurons and glia of the peripheral nervous system as well as of the melanocytes in the skin. This story is somewhat puzzling, García-Castro said, given that the neural crest cells also make many other derivatives in the cranial region that are normally associated with mesoderm. He questioned how a cell that is derived from the ectoderm could simultaneously generate all of the neural crest derivatives. This phenomenon is discordant with the Waddington's epigenetics and post gastrulation restrictions that suggest that mesoderm, ectoderm, and endoderm should only differentiate into derivatives of each lineage. "For an ectodermaly derived neural crest to generate a mesoderm derivative, it would have to bypass the ectoderm restriction, climb up a hill and go to the other valley," he remarked.

Ontogeny of Neural Crest

García-Castro's laboratory is using a variety of model organisms and model systems to revisit the ontogeny of neural crest cells and determine when those cells are specified.

Specification of Neural Crest Cell Fate

The perception that neural processes are specified in the ectoderm comes from a series of studies from the 1980s and 1990s, which showed that neural crest cells appear in between the neural and non-neural ectoderm. This suggests that those two tissues interact with mesoderm that lies underneath them, inducing the appearance of neural crest cells in a classical fashion. This is thought to be mediated by the BMP, fibroblast growth factors (FGFs), and Wnt pathways, among others, which lead to a cascade of transcription factors and other markers that are expressed at the neural plate border and are responsible for the development of neural crest cells. However, the work of García-Castro's laboratory suggests that the specification of these neural crest cells can actually be traced much earlier to the epiblast, before the definitive mesoderm and neural tissues appear. The researchers in García-Castro's laboratory have identified a specific region of the pre-gastrula epiblast with cells that are poised to make neural crest cells, although they do not express known markers. To frame his discussion, García-Castro defined the concept of specification in this context. Specification is the initiation of a program—in this case, the initiation of the neural crest cell fate program. The specified cell does not display known neural crest markers yet, but it is able to do so under "undisruptive" conditions. The researchers use the markers that are seen later on in neural crest cells to assess cell fate. This does not suggest that these cells are committed to form neural crest cells, García-Castro said; they are still plastic and can be persuaded to do otherwise in the embryo. In researching early avian neural crest development, García-Castro and colleagues identified the expression of Pax7 in a restricted region between the prospective neural plate and epidermis at the early stages of development. No other marker of the neural process is expressed in such a restricted fashion at this early stage, and it precedes the expression of later markers such as Snail2, SOX9, and Ets1. Inhibiting Pax7 blocked the expression of several of those markers, demonstrating that it was required for neural crest cells and further indicating that some cells are already specified in the embryo before they express Pax7 (Basch et al., 2006).

Blastula Studies of Neural Crest Cell Specification

García-Castro provided an overview of his laboratory's recent work on the specification of neural crest cells in chicks during the blastula stage. In the first phase, his team monitored for the expression of the Pax7 marker after dissecting epiblast tissues, explanting them into collagen gels, and culturing them in isolation under non-inductive conditions. A clear spatiotemporal restriction was observed between explants that can and cannot express Pax7, with Pax7 only appearing in the intermediate, not the center or the most lateral territories. After the explants had been incubated for a longer period, other neural crest markers emerged, and eventually the definitive markers of migratory neural crest cells were evident in the restricted intermediate territories. García-Castro and his colleagues followed up with a series of experiments to determine whether neural crest markers are induced in culture. First, they cut the explants and disassociated the cultures that were generating a low density of prospective neural crest cells—that is, the cells were not isolated, but they were far apart from each other. Then the researchers compared the explant from the central (control) territory with the explants from the lateral territory, which were cultured under the same conditions. At the time the explants were cut, the cells in the intermediate territory were already poised to express Pax7. After 25 hours, the researchers could identify cells that were clearly far away from each other in the large-volume culture, which makes it unlikely that the cells were responding to contact mediated signals from neighbors and induced in the classical way. These cells that were disassociated long before gastrulation at stage XII of embryonic development and cultured at low density went on to express Pax7 and SOX9, while those cultured from the central territory did not. A subsequent set of experiments looked at epiblast fate mapping by labeling cells in the epiblast with fluorescent dyes (DiI and DiO) and found that intermediate territories contributed to cells that go on to express Pax7 in the lateral territory that abuts the neural folds; the researchers also observed the label in the neural folds and migratory neural crest cells. Based on these findings, García-Castro and colleagues have built a map that shows the lateral region as containing prospective neural crest cells at these early stages of development. This is aligned with previous work suggesting that neural cells are specified in the center of the epiblast (Wilson et al., 2001).

Modeling Early Human Neural Crest Development with Pluripotent Stem Cells

Considering the question of whether human neural crest also specified before gastrulation and whether the knowledge gained from neural crest in chicks can be translated to humans, García-Castro said that knowledge of neural crest cell development in human embryos is still limited to histological descriptions of neural crest cells under migratory routes, with minimal molecular information available. To address this knowledge gap, García-Castro and colleagues obtained a collection of embryos and characterized a battery of markers expressed by human neural crest cells in pre-migratory or migratory states (Betters et al., 2010). However, this was not sufficient to determine whether specification was occurring at the very early stage, and those types of embryos are difficult to access. Thus, the researchers turned to modeling the development of human neural crest with PSCs, following work initiated by Pomp et al. (2005) and carried out in various other labs, and informed by the García-Castro lab's own work on neural crest cell development in the embryo. The researchers developed a system to rapidly derive human neural crest from hESCs via Wnt in defined media (Leung et al., 2016). Using low-density cultures of cells that display characteristics of stem cells but no neural crest cell markers, they observed robust expression of Pax7 and SOX10 in just 5 days. Ultimately, the model was used to show the expression of all neural crest cell markers of interest as well as to demonstrate the capacity to generate all of the neural crest cell derivatives that are expected from neural crest cells. This demonstrates that the Wnt-induced cells are bona fide neural crest cells, García-Castro said.

Advantages of the Model

García-Castro's model follows many others that have induced neural crest from hPSC (Chambers et al., 2013; Fukuta et al., 2014; Lee et al., 2007a; Menendez et al., 2011; Mica et al., 2013; Pomp et al., 2005). However, he said, his model is unique in several ways. It is the most rapid, and it is the only one that does not use either fading of serum replacement or TGF-beta inhibition. His team has used the model to characterize the signaling parameters of neural crest cell development, including the window of time of exposure for Wnt and the concentration of Wnt. Using the model, it is possible to modulate the identity of the neural crest cells and make neural crest derivatives according to the desired axial region—that is, higher levels of Wnt can make posterior neural crest cells and low levels of Wnt can make anterior neural crest cells (Gomez et al., 2019a,b). The protocol has also been modified to generate a robust platform that has high efficiency across multiple types of cells, including ESCs or induced pluripotent stem cells (Hackland et al., 2019). Furthermore, the model addresses the ontogeny of the neural crest cells by demonstrating—contrary to the prevailing model—that neither neural ectoderm nor mesoderm is required to form neural crest cells. Instead, the model holds that there is a very early lineage derived from the epiblast, which García-Castro calls "pre-border," that expresses specific markers that lead to neural crest cell formation. This holds specifically for early anterior neural crest cells, he noted. To further analyze the ontogeny of human neural crest cells, García-Castro's laboratory has looked at different characteristics of early induction in the epiblast using epigenetic, transcriptomic, and functional assays, including a comparison of the epigenetic regulation and expression of ESC and neural crest cell markers after Wnt induction. He and his colleagues have found that neural crest proteins are upregulated in prospective neural crest cells soon after Wnt activation, as indicated by the expression of neural crest markers (Leung et al., 2019). Additionally, functional assays suggest that 6 hours after exposure to Wnt, the cells have initiated the path to neural crest cell formation.

Early Neural Crest Cell Development in Mammals

Reflecting on how to translate gains from chick and model human neural crest studies to mammalian embryos in order to enable more robust comparisons, García-Castro said that much progress has been made using mouse models to study neural crest cells in the later stages of development, but little is known about how the neural crest cells are formed or specified (Murdoch et al., 2010, 2012). A challenge lies in rodent-specific pre-gastrula development. A chick embryo has a large territory that allows for high spatiotemporal resolution; the mouse embryo is very small in comparison, which makes it difficult to dissect effectively. Another issue is that the mouse embryo adopts a cup-like shape rather than lying flat, and the murine germ layers are inverted in early stages. This makes the mouse a less appropriate model for modeling neural crest cell development in a way that is informative for other mammals, including humans. Consequently,

García-Castro's laboratory is working to integrate the rabbit as a mammalian alternative model of neural crest cell development. The rabbit is larger than the mouse, allowing for better spatiotemporal resolution, and it has a flat blastodisk like the chick and human embryos. By characterizing neural crest development in very early stages in the rabbit, he and his colleagues have found the expression of mesoderm, neural, and neural crest markers. They identified Pax7 as the first restricted marker of neural crest cells as well as identifying several other NC markers, including SOX9 and SOX10, that have been shown in other model organisms. As shown in the mouse, they observed neural crest emigration before the tube closes. Most importantly, they found that rabbit neural crest cells are specified during gastrulation (Betters et al., 2018). For the first time in a mammal, they were able to dissect the epiblast of the gastrula embryo to generate and culture explants, demonstrating that although the intermediate territory is specified to form neural crest cells, it does not co-express mesoderm markers. Over time, they express crest markers, and they are subjected to signaling restrictions similar to those found in the chick.

BLASTOCYST-LIKE STRUCTURES GENERATED FROM PLURIPOTENT STEM CELLS WITH EXPANDED POTENTIAL

Jun Wu, an assistant professor of molecular biology at the University of Texas Southwestern Medical Center, explained how blastocyst-like structures (blastoids) can be generated from pluripotent stem cells systems in vitro in order to study early development. He described how the in vitro model mimics pre-implantation development in vivo and considered the development potential of these model structures in utero.

Building a Blastocyst-Like Structure Using Stem Cells

Describing the fundamentals of building a blastocyst-like structure using pluripotent stem cells, Wu explained that pluripotency is a continuum rather than a singular state of development (Graham and Zernicka-Goetz, 2016). To construct a blastocyst-like structure, the task is to select which type of pluripotent stem cells to use in order to adapt the in vivo continuum of pluripotency to an in vitro environment. Pluripotent stem cells can be generated by (1) isolating them from early embryos by taking out the ICM and then expanding them under different culture conditions or (2) inducing them from fibroblast and other somatic cells. Depending on when and what kind of cells are isolated, pluripotent cells have different properties. By developing different culture conditions, stem cells can be cultured in several different pluripotent states. The most well-known pluripotent states are naïve and primed. The naïve in vitro pluripotent state represents an earlier type of pluripotent stem cell in vivo, which is very similar to the epiblast of an E4.5 embryo. The prime pluripotent state represents a peri-gastrulation stage of the epiblast when it is primed for differentiation.

In order to generate a blastocyst-like structure, the naïve pluripotent stem cell would seem to be the logical choice, Wu said; however, the blastocyst contains more than one cell type, so generating a blastocyst requires at least two to three different types of cells. Over the past several decades, three stem cell lines have been generated: trophoblast stem cells (TSCs) (Tanaka et al., 1998), extraembryonic endoderm (XEN) stem cells (Kunath et al., 2005), and ESCs (Evans and Kaufman, 1981; Martin, 1981). Rivron has demonstrated that aggregating TSCs and ESCs in culture can generate a blastoid structure, which looks like a blastocyst and expresses several blastocyst markers (Rivron et al., 2018b). Several years ago another type of pluripotent stem cell was derived from early embryos, called extended- or expanded-potential pluripotent stem cells (EPSCs) (Yang et al., 2017a,b). These cells can generate both embryonic and extraembryonic lineages, such as placenta and yolk sac. A single EPSC injected into an 8-cell stage embryo can contribute to both the trophectoderm and the ICM of a blastocyst.

Building a Blastocyst-Like Structure from Expanded-Potential Pluripotent Stem Cells

Wu and colleagues looked at whether EPSCs can self-organize to generate a blastocyst-like structure (blastoid) in culture (Li et al., 2019). Figure 5-1 depicts an overview of the process. After aggregating four to five EPSCs under the appropriate conditions for 4–6 days, the cells differentiated and self-organized into a blastoid-like structure, which Wu's team named an "EPS-blastoid." Initially, the cells formed a cluster without distinct morphology, but after a few days, a blastocyst-like cavity and an ICM-like structure began to form. Visual comparison revealed that the EPS-blastoid looked similar to a blastocyst isolated from an in vivo E3.5 stage embryo. Using two different cell lines, they found that about 15 percent of the structures looked like blastocysts, but the other structures were disorganized and showed markers in different locations.

First Cell Fate Determination in EPS-Blastoids: Trophectoderm and Inner Cell Mass

To further characterize the EPS-blastoid, Wu and colleagues looked first at the expression of two transcription factors that are characteristic of the trophectoderm (TE) and the ICM: CDX2 and SOX2. CDX2 was expressed in the outer layer of the cells of the blastoid, while SOX2 was localized to

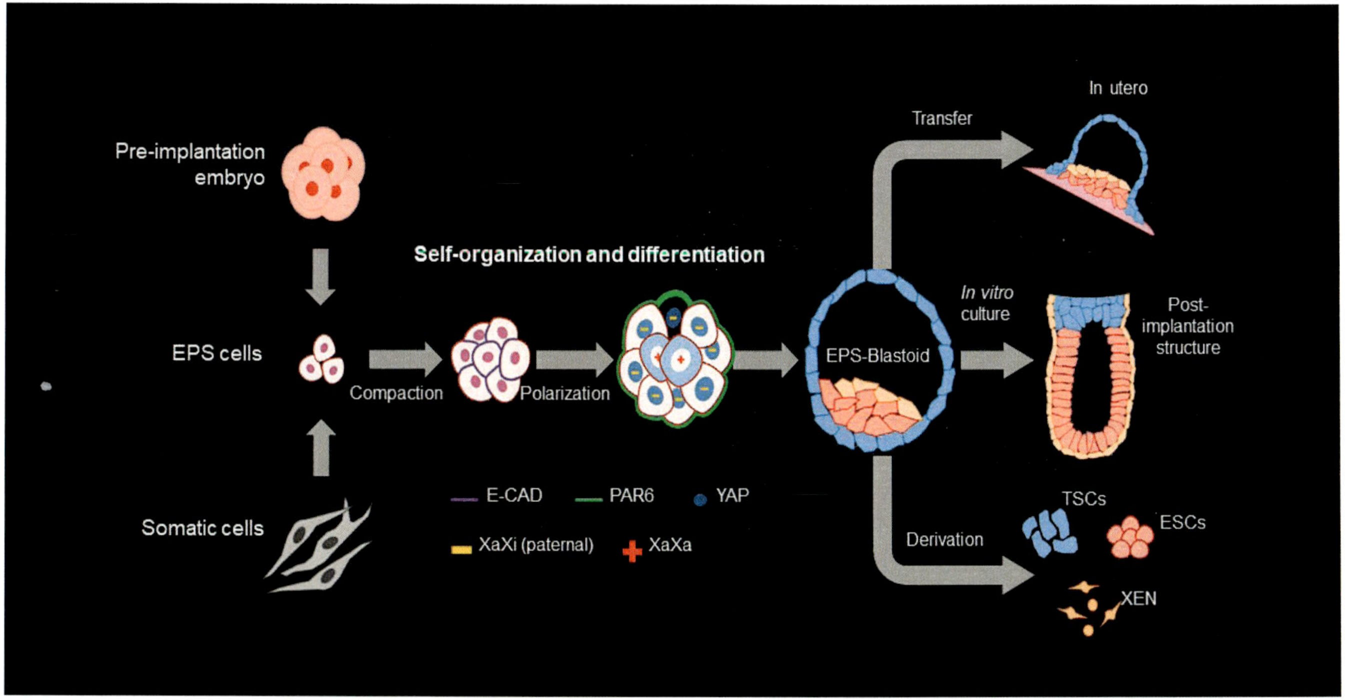

FIGURE 5-1 Blastocyst-like structure generated in vitro using expanded- or extended-potential stem cells.
NOTE: EPS = expanded-potential stem; ESC = embryonic stem cell; TSC = trophoblast stem cell; XEN = extraembryonic endoderm.
SOURCES: Jun Wu workshop presentation, January 17, 2020.

the ICM. This suggested that at least the first cell fate commitment in some of the structure had been made. In about 75 percent of the aggregates, the inside cells expressed SOX2, NANOG, or OCT4, and the outside cells expressed CDX2. However, other structures were generated that did not appear like blastocysts. To further investigate, the researchers counted the numbers of cells in the ICM and TE. At day 6, the numbers of both the CDX2-positive cells and the SOX2-positive cells were comparable to a blastocyst isolated in vivo.

Second Cell Fate Determination in EPS-Blastoids: Epiblast and Primitive Endoderm

Next, Wu and colleagues looked at whether EPS-blastoids could further develop into structures resembling a mature blastocyst, which contains three cell lineages instead of two. In some of the EPS-blastoids, they observed that some inside cells expressed GATA4, a marker of the primitive endoderm (PE) while other inside cells expressed NANOG. This suggested that the second cell fate determination had also occurred in some of the structures. However, the efficiency was low, with only 20 percent of the EPS-blastoids actually giving rise to a mature blastocyst-like structure containing all three cell lineages. The numbers of cells in the structures were comparable to those in a mature blastocyst at the E4.5 stage, with both NANOG-positive cells and GATA4-positive cells coming from the epiblast and primitive endoderm lineages.

Transcriptomic Features of EPS-Blastoids

A global transcriptome analysis was performed to identify transcriptomic features of EPS-blastoids, Wu said. First, they used bulk RNA sequencing to compare the EPS-blastoid with natural blastocysts and morulae. It appeared as though the blastoid they generated was closer to a blastocyst than a morula, suggesting that the EPS-blastoid was more like a 3.5-day blastocyst than a 2.5-day morula embryo. Single-cell RNA-sequencing analysis confirmed that all three cell lineages in the EPS-blastoid had been properly segregated. Of interest, the researchers observed that many cells that were intermediate between the epiblasts and trophectoderm, suggesting that the first cell commitment in some of the aggregates was not properly allocated.

EPS-Blastoid Formation Mimics Pre-Implantation Development

Wu and colleagues then looked at whether the system for EPS-blastoid formation could be used to model pre-implantation development (Ramanujam et al., 2017). Several morphological and molecular processes occur during pre-implantation development, he said, including compaction, polarization, differential yes-associated protein (YAP) localization in the TE and ICM compartments, and X chromosome inactivation in the trophectoderm layer via preferential silencing of the X chromosome from the paternal side. He and his colleagues observed compaction occurring as early as day 1 as well as polarization occurring during blastoid formation. Looking at Hippo–YAP signaling in the outer layer cells of the trophectoderm, they saw most of YAP localized to the nucleus. However, in the ICM there was a diffused staining of YAP. Wu said that they used an inhibitor of YAP that was effective in stalling mouse embryo development, so the EPSC aggregates failed to form any blastoid-type structures in the presence of that inhibitor. He and his colleagues observed that in about 80 percent of the structures, the TE-like layer preferentially silenced the X chromosome from the paternal side. A functional test of the EPS-blastoid was whether it could be used to derive all three types of stem cells, Wu said. And, indeed, using the EPS-blastoid, they were able to derive all three types: (1) ESCs, which gave rise to adult chimeras, (2) TSCs, which could contribute to placenta tissue, and (3) XEN cells, which contributed to the yolk sac membrane after injection into the blastocyst.

Developmental Potential of EPS-Blastoids Post-Implantation and In Utero

The next step was to culture the EPS-blastoid in vitro to post-implantation-like structure, which they performed using the culture protocol developed by Zernicka-Goetz (Bedzhov et al., 2014). During this extended culture of the EPS-blastoid, they observed morphogenic events that modeled peri- and post-implantation development. In some of the structures the epiblast became polarized by day 3 and pro-amniotic cavities started to form by day 5. However, the efficiency decreased dramatically the longer they were cultured in vitro. To explore the in utero developmental potential of EPS-blastoids, they transferred them into the uterus and observed implantation. Some of the deciduae generated by the EPS-blastoid were similar in size to an in vivo decidua, and markers for EPI, TE, and PE were expressed in some of the structures' cells. However, the structures were malformed, disorganized, and abnormal compared with the normal development of an embryo after transplantation into the uterus. He and his colleagues have also been able to derive and implant blastoids using iPS-cell-derived EPSCs, he added, which were generated with similar efficiency, as would be expected from EPSCs derived from embryos.

Use of Human Expanded-Potential Stem Cells

In addition to the mouse studies, two studies have shown that human EPSCs can be derived from the early embryo or induced from somatic cells (Gao et al., 2019; Yang et al., 2017b). Injecting a single human EPSC can contribute to the TE and ICM compartments in a mouse blastocyst, but it is inefficient for generating any type of blastocyst-like structure. Although some of the structures look similar to a natural human blastocyst, after staining the proper markers are not expressed in the right locations. "It's safe to say that, using the mouse protocol, we haven't been able to generate similar structures from human EPSCs that resemble a human blastocyst," Wu said.

PANEL DISCUSSION

Use of Human Expanded-Potential Stem Cells in Mouse Models

Why do hEPSCs not appear to work as well as mouse EPSCs in the model produced by Wu's team? one workshop participant asked. Wu offered several reasons why his team did not observe successful formation of the human blastoid from EPSCs: (1) EPS culture conditions and cell quality are different for human and mouse, and blastocyst-like structures could be generated from early but not late passage human EPSCs; (2) species differences between human and mouse during early development may also play a role, for example, if the two species differ in the timing of TE, EPI, and PE lineage specifications; and (3) the protocol used for generating blastoids from mouse EPSCs is not necessarily applicable to humans. The success in generating the mouse EPS-blastoid relied on an initial biased differentiation toward the TE lineage, Wu said. In the mouse, adding in factors like FGF4 or Wnt agonist can promote TE differentiation of the EPS cells. However, the signals that promote the human TE differentiation from human EPS cells remain unknown.

Impact of Chromosomal Disruption on Fertility

What is the impact of chromosomal disruption on human infertility, a workshop participant asked, and are there implications for pre-implantation diagnosis? The participant noted that cows are highly fertile, but the degree of chromosomal disruption in cows is comparable to that in humans. The use of nonhuman primate studies can help shed light on this issue, Chavez said, adding that when she and her colleagues investigated this in the time-mated breeding colony at their primate center, they found that 74 percent (the same percentage of rhesus cleavage-stage embryos that were aneuploid to some degree) of the confirmed ovulation and mating cases did not result in a live birth. Thus, only about 30 percent of those resulted in a live birth, which is relatively similar to what is seen in humans. The impact of in vitro versus in vivo maturation of oocytes is a relevant consideration for cows, she added. However, a comparison between bovine embryos derived in vivo and in vitro revealed an aneuploidy rate of 18 percent even in the embryos derived in vivo.

Fragmentation in Aneuploid Embryos

In response to a question about whether all aneuploid embryos appear to fragment, Chavez replied that this question has persisted for decades. In fact, clinicians used to remove fragments because they thought it would improve the embryo. Her group's working hypothesis is that fragmentation is an inefficient process that is a response to micronucleation. Fragmented embryos have yet to be observed in any species that does not also have micronuclei formation, which suggests that fragmentation will not occur without aneuploidy. These observations are based on recapitulation in the nonhuman primate, she said, and it may not be possible to study this in humans. It is challenging to study maternal-age-related aneuploidy in nonhuman primates, she added, because most of their monkeys are relatively young. Thus, they observe fewer meiotic errors than in a typical human IVF population. The invasive primitive in situ trophoblast does not seem to be an extensive population in monkeys, Golos said. Rather than invasion, there is more of an expansive proliferation of a trophoblastic cell. Although there are pockets of in situ trophoblasts, they do not intrude substantially into the decidua, as the human embryo does. This suggests that nonhuman primates may not provide the best model for understanding the earliest events contributing to the high rate of implantation failure in human embryos, he said. Much of this increased aneuploidy might be driven by recombination rates, which vary across species, a participant said.

Alternative Nonhuman Primate Models

Golos and Chavez were asked whether nonhuman primates that are closer to humans than macaques would be more useful systems for modeling in certain situations. Access to more closely related nonhuman primates would be challenging, Golos said, but iPS cells might offer an alternative. Marmosets are also an option, but marmoset embryology is even more different from humans than macaque embryology. Chavez replied that at her primate center they have cynomolgus macaques (cynos), rhesus macaques, baboons, and marmosets. Baboons are primarily used for contraceptive studies. Gibbons have an interesting genome for study, but they are protected as an endangered species. Cynos have the advantage of being non-seasonal breeders, while rhesus have a decline in oocyte quality during the summer months.

Improvement of In Vitro Fertilization Culture Conditions

Chavez was asked about the percentage of aneuploid embryos in IVF that arise from meiosis versus mitosis and if cultures and protocols might be altered to either prevent aneuploidy from occurring or encourage its correction. Meiotic errors are more common in older women, Chavez said, but her group has intentionally tried to look at younger women to obtain a better assessment of error types and frequencies. She added that she is particularly interested in studying embryos that have a meiotic error and that then have a greater propensity to have a mitotic error. She said that she is often asked whether aneuploidy is a consequence of in vitro culture. Although this is difficult to study in humans, the phenomenon of cellular fragmentation is highly associated with aneuploidy and occurs in vivo in humans and many other species. Culture conditions could still probably be improved for humans and other mammals, she added.

Metabolic Stress and Culture Conditions

A participant commented that research comparing cortical organoids from humans to primary data have revealed gene differences related to metabolic stress across all of the published protocols, indicating that culture conditions somehow create metabolic stress. Correcting for metabolic stress eliminated the abnormal gene expression in the cortical organoids, and the fidelity of the model improved. The participant suggested that it might also hold true for the iPS of the stem cell–derived blastocyst and perhaps even in the IVF clinic. If so, it might be possible to correct for this and improve culture conditions. Wu remarked that when culturing pluripotent cells, the cells are removed from the early embryo and placed in a culture condition that is very different from the in vivo environment. In human naïve-like embryonic stem cells or iPS cells that have been generated, defects have been observed in imprinting status, and if cultured long enough, metabolic defects would likely also be observed. The cells also accumulate genomic instabilities and karyotypical abnormalities after long-term culture. Better culture conditions that more closely mimic the in vivo environment could enable cells to grow and differentiate more naturally. However, comparing transcriptomes from pluripotent stem cells cultured in vitro to in vivo embryos shows that in vitro cultured cells always cluster together and separate from in vivo counterparts, regardless of the culture conditions used. This suggests that there are some in vivo features that have not yet been recapitulated in vitro. Although some features can be preserved in pluripotent stem cell cultures (e.g., mouse ESCs can generate chimera similar to the early epiblast) other features differ between in vivo and in vitro, such as metabolic and epigenetic features. Chavez added that an ongoing metabolomics analysis of monkey oocytes fertilized in culture from which the spent culture media was obtained indicates that stress may actually be set up even in the oocyte. The glucocorticoid pathway is one of the main signaling pathways observed in oocytes that go on to fertilize, cleave, and progress to the blastocyst stage. She noted that people often assume that stress experienced by a woman is the cause of oocyte difficulties. However, her group is finding that the systemic level of metabolites appears to be quite different than the levels in the follicular environment, underscoring the importance of good starting material. "If we do not have a good egg to begin with, we are probably not going to have a good embryo," she said. Golos noted that extended culture experiments are typically performed in 20 percent oxygen, which is not the natural environment for an embryo or trophoblast. Chavez added that according to probe studies in the monkey, oxygen concentration is only about 1 percent even in the ovary, suggesting that culturing should be performed in low oxygen.

6

Exploring Opportunities and Challenges with Mammalian Embryo Model Systems

The final session of the workshop featured a closing keynote lecture from Martin Pera and a panel discussion focused on future opportunities and challenges with mammalian embryo model systems. Panelists were asked to summarize the lessons learned and the topics discussed throughout the workshop. They also considered novel strategies that could be moved forward to help advance the field and the level of fidelity that exists between model systems of human embryos and bona fide human embryos. The session was moderated by Nicolas Rivron. The final panel discussion included Ali Brivanlou, Jianping Fu, Kathy Niakan, and Mana Parast. Janet Rossant delivered closing remarks to wrap up the workshop.

HUMAN PLURIPOTENT STEM CELLS, THE HUMAN EMBRYO, AND THE SELF-RENEWING STATE

In his closing keynote lecture, M. Pera explored the developmental status of human pluripotent cells. Two fundamental questions about embryo models that remain unanswered were highlighted: the developmental status of human pluripotent stem cells and the stage of mammalian development that these cells most closely resemble. Understanding pluripotent cells in a developmental context is important for (1) comparative studies of early development, (2) the use of those cells as models of human embryonic development, and (3) understanding how best to direct lineage specification and differentiation, M. Pera said. Furthermore, it is not clear whether work on developing embryo models is starting with cells at the optimal pluripotent state or whether these cells are epigenetically or otherwise off-center.

The current understanding of the various states of cell pluripotency is largely based on work in the mouse, M. Pera said. Mouse naïve cells are embryonic stem cells (ESCs) maintained under conditions that strongly suppress differentiation (E4.5 epiblast). Epiblast stem cells (EpiSCs) correspond to late primitive streak stage (E7.5), which is almost the last stage in which pluripotent cells are seen in the embryo. Epiblast-like stem cells are an unstable cell type that corresponds to formative pluripotency in the early post-implantation epiblast (E5.5). These are naïve cells that have gone through a transition that then enables them to respond to the signals that will drive lineage specification. The naïve state, or ground state, is a stage in embryonic development at which the pluripotent cells are capable of forming all somatic tissues and the germ line and are lacking in any bias toward differentiation into any particular fate in the pre-implantation epiblast. This state can be maintained in vitro by strong pharmacologic blockade of signaling pathways that drive differentiation. In a mouse, only naïve pluripotent cells are capable of generating germ line chimeras. Mouse EpiSCs correspond to the late gastrula-stage embryo and show lineage priming (i.e., co-expression of pluripotency genes along the lineage-specific genes), M. Pera said (Kojima et al., 2014).

There have been some attempts to create human naïve cells, M. Pera said. Human ESCs and induced pluripotent stem cells (iPSCs) resemble in some respects mouse EpiSCs, but not mouse ESCs, and human ESCs and iPSCs are widely considered to be equivalent to them. However, this interpretation is based on relatively limited interspecies comparative data and does not take into account heterogeneity in stem cell populations. Human naïve PSCs equivalent to mouse naïve cells have not yet been described, though some cell lines similar to human pre-implantation epiblast have been developed. The maintenance of genetically stable human naïve PSCs has proven problematic, and mouse naïve cells may be epigenetically unstable under some conditions. The embryonic equivalent of the stable attractor state represented by human lines and conventional lines remains unknown, M. Pera said. He calls this a "stable attractor" state because regardless of whether the lines are made from the human teratocarcinoma, an embryo, or from reprogramming, under a wide range of culture conditions they revert and settle into this particular state, which is the conventional human stem cell. Assessment of the developmental status of human pluripotent cells is complicated by heterogeneity in cultures, as it was originally in the mouse, and there are subpopulations of pluripotent cells within the human cultures with distinct biological properties and gene expression (Kolle et al., 2009; Laslett et al., 2007). Only a minority of the cells in human PSC cultures show a high capacity for self-renewal.

Human pluripotent stem cells grown in the conventional fashion that have a high capacity for self-renewal also have a metabolic and cell cycle status similar to the mouse peri-implantation epiblast, M. Pera said. Transcriptionally, conventional hPSCs with high self-renewal capacity correspond most nearly to peri-implantation primate epiblast (E13–E16). In terms of development capacity, conventional hPSCs with high self-renewal capcity are competent to give rise to germ line cells similar to early post-implantation mouse epiblast formative cells. Self-renewing hPSCs do not resemble mouse epiblast stem cells and are not primed for any particular fate, he added. When the embryo implants in the mouse, the epiblast cells are no longer capable of differentiating to extraembryonic trophoblast or primitive endoderm. Whether the same developmental restriction occurs in the primate is unclear. Several other questions that remain to be addressed include will clonal growth and genetic stability improve if it is possible to maintain self-renewing subpopulations of hPSCs in pure form in culture. Much of the variation in the differentiation capacity of iPSC lines is genetically determined by the background of the donor. However, it is yet unknown if the variation in the differentiation capacity of hPSC lines arises from variation in the stability of substrates within the cultures.

FINAL PANEL DISCUSSION

Fidelity of Model Systems

Stem cells have been used to form different embryo models that recapitulate specific windows of development, Rivron said. However, these models are still crude in that they only recapitulate certain features of development rather than capturing the entire process. He asked the panelists to comment about the fidelity of the models presented (i.e., the extent to which they represent what they are intended to model) and about how those models could be made more reliable. For models of the earliest stages of development, questions of fidelity are among the most challenging to answer, Brivanlou said. Assessing fidelity for his models would require specimens that are samples of normal human development post-attachment, which are not accessible. The best option is to morphologically compare a given state of embryogenesis with the limited number of pictures that are available from the Carnegie or Kyoto embryo collections.[1] Another barrier to evaluating the fidelity of his models, Brivanlou said, is the lack

[1]More information about the Carnegie Institution of Washington's collection of human embryos can be found at https://embryo.asu.edu/pages/carnegie-institution-washington-department-embryology (accessed April 2, 2020), and for a more detailed history of the Kyoto Collection of Human Embryos and Fetuses, see Yamaguchi and Yamada (2018).

of control over the genetic backgrounds of his specimens or other variables based on ethnicity, diet, and metabolism, for example. Rivron observed that benchmarks are needed to understand what happens in real human embryos so those benchmarks can be used to verify these models. Studying human embryos is also important in order to examine the genetic variability that naturally occurs in humans but is poorly recapitulated in stem cells, Rivron added.

Advantages of Modeling Across Species

There is room for improvement in prolonging in vitro culture of human and nonhuman primate embryos, Fu said. He suggested that, in principle, nonhuman primate embryos could be cultured to establish benchmarks for calibrating in vitro human stem cell models. Golos suggested analyzing archived material from nonhuman primates for markers that are being discovered in extended culture or pluripotent cell studies. He also suggested that extended culture of nonhuman primate embryos has great potential to complement human studies, and he noted that in the past, human advances such as in vitro fertilization have been translated to the nonhuman primate. There are approaches in human embryology that can be complemented by applying human advances to other species, Brivanlou said, and creating this type of feedback loop may help to further our understanding of human embryology. This will require improving the comparative ability to interpret human development based on what is thought to occur in other systems, he said. Furthermore, a limitation that transcends the human system and affects all embryogenesis is the existence of critical dimensions and variables that are being missed in current measurements. For example, Brivanlou said, simple factors heretofore unconsidered (e.g., contour, mechanical forces, tissue stiffness) are now emerging as major instructive factors in guiding cell fate, path information, and morphogenesis. Model systems are useful in uncovering these types of new dimensions in other species and applying them to study human origins in particular, and embryology more broadly. It would be a mistake to consider all nonhuman primates together, Parast said. Many species have yet to be studied, and it is likely that some will be better than others in recapitulating different elements, such as placentation or trophoblast differentiation of the pluripotent stem cell, she said.

Open Questions with Embryonic Development

Despite progress in understanding development in general, large mysteries remain, Renee Reijo Pera said. Brivanlou's philosophical perspective is that everything is a cycle within a cycle: the union of the sperm and egg gives rise to an adult who produces sperm and eggs that give rise to another adult. Similarly, generating a model of human embryos began by using ESCs, which themselves came from an inner cell mass of a blastocyst. In that sense, it is almost like sending the human ESCs "back home" when they are put into the three-dimensional (3D) context of an embryo. "The fact that this very strong aspect of self-assembly and self-organization seems to be the driving force behind that, is not only mysterious, but also really beautiful," Brivanlou said, "and there is something in there that is beyond our scientific measurements and evaluations."

Fidelity of Three-Dimensional Systems

M. Pera asked the panelists about the extent to which 3D systems—which are presumed to be closer to normal embryonic conditions—are actually better in terms of fidelity or function than previous, cruder approaches. This gets close to the contentious question of whether researchers make models that are better than the original, Brivanlou said. Creating a model that is better than reality could be advantageous, for example, if it fixed something that is aberrant (e.g., curing a disease) in a way that is not otherwise possible. The issue is much more complicated in borderline cases, he said. Brivanlou went on to question the extent to which human or primate embryological work can be rationalized or justified based on utilitarian grounds versus the desire for basic knowledge. In his experience, he said, support and funding are not generally forthcoming in response to arguments based on the need to understand our human origins; utilitarian arguments based on the potential to cure disease, for example, tend to be more effective.

Further investment is needed to characterize the basics of early development across many species, including humans, Niakan said. Fundamental mechanisms of the earliest stages of human development are only beginning to be elucidated, but knowledge about the extent to which these mechanisms are conserved across species is needed before they can be recapitulated in vitro, she said. That knowledge will also be required to make improvements to directed-differentiation protocols that will be needed to make cells of potential therapeutic relevance and start to accurately model diseases. In many directed-differentiation protocols, the cell types produced are early precursor progenitor cells and not the mature cells that are needed, she said. Her philosophy is that "one never knows what will ultimately arise from all of that knowledge, but the knowledge itself is extremely important."

Contribution of Model Systems

The epigenetic status of human systems (e.g., variable methylation) is a complicating factor, M. Pera said, and it might be rectified by culturing cells in more natural conditions. Rather than trying to identify or generate better cells, Fu said his group is trying to develop model systems that allow for obtaining embryonic antigen-like cells in 3D culture systems. That knowledge could then be used to understand how, in the human context, embryonic ectoderm drives epiblast gastrulation and primordial germ cells develop in the embryonic ectoderm compartment. Synthetic models provide experimental systems for studying those fundamental biological questions, which was not possible in the past, Fu said. Further novel and important uses for these systems are to study human placentation, miscarriage, and later complications of pregnancy, such as fetal growth restriction and preeclampsia, Parast added. She noted that this area of research has been underfunded and overlooked—in part because it is considered controversial. However, she suggested that framing this research in the context of improving pregnancy outcomes and improving life for the next generation could help demonstrate the importance of this type of work.

USING EMBRYO MODELS TO UNDERSTAND HUMAN DEVELOPMENT

In addition to understanding infertility, early embryo loss, and birth defects, M. Pera suggested that investigating the embryonic origins of adult diseases is another important rationale for studying the human embryo. This is a controversial area of research, he said, but evidence suggests that epigenetic programming during early development affects the onset of disease in later life, particularly cardiometabolic and neurological disorders. Embryo systems could be used to address these issues, he suggested, as well as to provide opportunities to improve the fidelity of stem cell differentiation. Two decades ago, when his laboratory and others first started to derive cell lines from the human blastocyst, they were asked to justify the use of human embryos in this research, M. Pera said. In Australia, the question was not whether researchers would be funded by the government to do this research; the question was whether they would be put in jail for doing it, he said. One of the arguments researchers there made was that embryo systems would ultimately be useful for informing the understanding of human development, and based on what he heard during the workshop, he said, the prospects for achieving that have never been better.

In her final remarks, Rossant underscored the wealth of opportunities that are now available to study human development in new ways using actual human embryos and stem cell models in culture systems. However, progress remains to be made to understand enough about the early human embryo to establish benchmarks and comparators. Regarding stem cells themselves, much remains to be understood about the state of those cells and how to maintain those states in the desired way. "We are not making human embryos in a dish; we are not making test tube babies; we are not generating anything that could in any way be considered as viable human embryos, nor is that the intent of the any of the research that you heard about today," Rossant emphasized. Instead, the aim is to study the important phases of human development that are relevant to issues of human infertility, placental problems, and disease. Embryo model systems provide a tremendous opportunity, she said, to better understand human development and to develop new tools to study disease.

References

Aldeguer, J. F., M. Kip, J. Vivie, L. Li, A. Alemany, J. Korving, F. Darmis, A. van Oudenaarden, N. Geijsen, and N. C. Rivron. 2019. Embryonic signals perpetuate polar-like trophoblast stem cells and pattern the blastocyst axis. *bioRxiv* 510362.

Alikani, M., J. Cohen, G. Tomkin, G. J. Garrisi, C. Mack, and R. T. Scott. 1999. Human embryo fragmentation in vitro and its implications for pregnancy and implantation. *Fertility and Sterility* 71(5):836–842.

Anderson, K. G., W. B. Hamilton, F. V. Roske, A. Azad, T. E. Knudsen, M. A. Canham, L. M. Forrester, and J. M. Brickman. 2017. Insulin fine-tunes self-renewal pathways governing naïve pluripotency and extra-embryonic endoderm. *Nature Cell Biology* 19(10):1164–1177.

Antczak, M., and J. Van Blerkom. 1999. Temporal and spatial aspects of fragmentation in early human embryos: Possible effects on developmental competence and association with the differential elimination of regulatory proteins from polarized domains. *Human Reproduction* 14(2):429–447.

Basch, M. L., M. Bronner-Fraser, and M. I. García-Castro. 2006. Specification of the neural crest occurs during gastrulation and requires Pax7. *Nature* 441(7090):218–222.

Bedzhov, I., and M. Zernicka-Goetz. 2014. Self-organizing properties of mouse pluripotent cells initiate morphogenesis upon implantation. *Cell* 156(5):1032–1044.

Bedzhov, I., C. Y. Leung, M. Bialecka, and M. Zernicka-Goetz. 2014. In vitro culture of mouse blastocysts beyond the implantation stages. *Nature Protocols* 9(12):2732–2739.

Betters, E., Y. Liu, A. Kjaeldgaard, E. Sundström, and M. I. García-Castro. 2010. Analysis of early human neural crest development. *Developmental Biology* 344(2):578–592.

Betters, E., R. M. Charney, and M. I. García-Castro. 2018. Early specification and development of rabbit neural crest cells. *Developmental Biology* 444:S181–S192.

Blaise, S., N. de Parseval, and T. Heidmann. 2005. Functional characterization of two newly identified human endogenous retrovirus coding envelope genes. *Retrovirology* 2:19.

Blakeley, P., N. M. Fogarty, I. Del Valle, S. E. Wamaitha, T. X. Hu, K. Elder, P. Snell, L. Christie, P. Robson, and K. K. Niakan. 2015. Defining the three cell lineages of the human blastocyst by single-cell RNA-seq. *Development* 142(18):3151–3165.

Bolton, H., S. J. L. Graham, N. Van der Aa, P. Kumar, K. Theunis, E. Fernandez Gallardo, T. Voet, and M. Zernicka-Goetz. 2016. Mouse model of chromosome mosaicism reveals lineage-specific depletion of aneuploid cells and normal developmental potential. *Nature Communications* 7:11165.

Boyd, J. D., and W. J. Hamilton. 1966. Electron microscopic observations on the cytotrophoblast contribution to the syncytium in the human placenta. *Journal of Anatomy* 100(Pt 3):535–548.

Britton, G., I. Heemskerk, R. Hodge, A. A. Qutub, and A. Warmflash. 2019. A novel self-organizing embryonic stem cell system reveals signaling logic underlying the patterning of human ectoderm. *Development* 146(20):dev179093.

Brons, I. G. M., L. E. Smithers, M. W. B. Trotter, P. Rugg-Gunn, B. Sun, S. M. C. de Sousa Lopes, S. K. Howlett, A. Clarkson, L. Ahrlund-Richter, R. A. Pedersen, and L. Vallier. 2007. Derivation of pluripotent epiblast stem cells from mammalian embryos. *Nature* 448(7150):191–195.

Brooks, K. E., B. L. Daughtry, E. Metcalf, K. Masterson, D. Battaglia, L. Gao, B. Park, and S. L. Chavez. 2019. Assessing equine embryo developmental competency by time-lapse image analysis. *Reproduction, Fertility, and Development* 31(12):1840–1850.

Buster, J. E., M. Bustillo, I. A. Rodi, S. W. Cohen, M. Hamilton, J. A. Simon, I. H. Thorneycroft, and J. R. Marshall. 1985. Biologic and morphologic development of donated human ova recovered by nonsurgical uterine lavage. *American Journal of Obstetrics and Gynecology* 153(2):211–217.

Chambers, S. M., Y. Mica, G. Lee, L. Studer, and M. J. Tomishima. 2013. Dual-SMAD Inhibition/WNT Activation-Based Methods to Induce Neural Crest and Derivatives from Human Pluripotent Stem Cells. *Human Embryonic Stem Cell Protocols* 1307:239–343.

Chang, T. A., G. I. Bondarenko, B. Gerami-Naini, J. G. Drenzek, M. Durning, M. A. Garthwaite, J. K. Schmidt, T. G. Golos, T. G. Golos, T. G. Golos, T. A. Chang, G. I. Bondarenko, B. Gerami-Naini, and J. G. Drenzek. 2018. Trophoblast differentiation, invasion and hormone secretion in a three-dimensional in vitro implantation model with rhesus monkey embryos. *Reproductive Biology and Endocrinology* 16(1):24.

Chavez, S. L., K. E. Loewke, J. Han, F. Moussavi, P. Colls, S. Munne, B. Behr, and R. A. Reijo Pera. 2012. Dynamic blastomere behaviour reflects human embryo ploidy by the four-cell stage. *Nature Communications* 3:1251.

Chavez, S. L., S. L. McElroy, N. L. Bossert, C. J. De Jonge, M. V. Rodriguez, D. E. Leong, B. Behr, L. M. Westphal, and R. A. Reijo Pera. 2014. Comparison of epigenetic mediator expression and function in mouse and human embryonic blastomeres. *Human Molecular Genetics* 23(18):4970–4984.

Chhabra, S., L. Liu, R. Goh, X. Kong, and A. Warmflash. 2019. Dissecting the dynamics of signaling events in the BMP, WNT, and NODAL cascade during self-organized fate patterning in human gastruloids. *PLOS Biology* 17(10):e3000498.

Chow, J. F. C., W. S. B. Yeung, E. Y. L. Lau, V. C. Y. Lee, E. H. Y. Ng, and P.-C. Ho. 2014. Array comparative genomic hybridization analyses of all blastomeres of a cohort of embryos from young IVF patients revealed significant contribution of mitotic errors to embryo mosaicism at the cleavage stage. *Reproductive Biology and Endocrinology* 12(1):105.

Crasta, K., N. J. Ganem, R. Dagher, A. B. Lantermann, E. V. Ivanova, Y. Pan, L. Nezi, A. Protopopov, D. Chowdhury, and D. Pellman. 2012. DNA breaks and chromosome pulverization from errors in mitosis. *Nature* 482(7383):53–58.

Daughtry, B. L., J. L. Rosenkrantz, N. Redmayne, S. L. Chavez, J. L. Rosenkrantz, K. A. Torkenczy, A. Adey, L. Carbone, N. H. Lazar, L. Carbone, S. S. Fei, M. Yan, L. Gao, B. Park, L. Carbone, A. Adey, K. A. Nevonen, L. Carbone, and S. L. Chavez. 2019. Single-cell sequencing of primate preimplantation embryos reveals chromosome elimination via cellular fragmentation and blastomere exclusion. *Genome Research* 29(3):367–382.

De Paepe, C., G. Cauffman, A. Verloes, J. Sterckx, P. Devroey, H. Tournaye, I. Liebaers, and H. Van de Velde. 2013. Human trophectoderm cells are not yet committed. *Human Reproduction (Oxford, England)* 28(3):740–749.

Deglincerti, A., G. F. Croft, L. N. Pietila, M. Zernicka-Goetz, E. D. Siggia, and A. H. Brivanlou. 2016. Self-organization of the in vitro attached human embryo. *Nature* 533(7602):251–254.

Destouni, A., M. Zamani Esteki, M. Catteeuw, O. Tsuiko, E. Dimitriadou, K. Smits, A. Kurg, A. Salumets, A. Van Soom, T. Voet, and J. R. Vermeesch. 2016. Zygotes segregate entire parental genomes in distinct blastomere lineages causing cleavage-stage chimerism and mixoploidy. *Genome Research* 26(5):567–578.

Dong, C., M. Beltcheva, P. Gontarz, B. Zhang, P. Popli, L. A. Fischer, S. A. Khan, K. M. Park, E. J. Yoon, X. Xing, R. Kommagani, T. Wang, L. Solnica-Krezel, and T. W. Theunissen. 2020. Derivation of trophoblast stem cells from naïve human pluripotent stem cells. *Elife* 9:e52504.

Dozortsev, D., A. Ermilov, D. M. El-Mowafi, and M. Diamond. 1998. The impact of cellular fragmentation induced experimentally at different stages of mouse preimplantation development. *Human Reproduction* 13(5):1307–1311.

Etoc, F., J. Metzger, A. Ruzo, C. Kirst, A. Yoney, M. Z. Ozair, A. H. Brivanlou, and E. D. Siggia. 2016. A balance between secreted inhibitors and edge-sensing controls gastruloid self-organization. *Developmental Cell* 39(3):302–315.

Evans, M. J., and M. H. Kaufman. 1981. Establishment in culture of pluripotential cells from mouse embryos. *Nature* 292(5819):154–156.

Fogarty, N. M. E., A. McCarthy, K. E. Snijders, B. E. Powell, N. Kubikova, P. Blakeley, R. Lea, K. Elder, S. E. Wamaitha, D. Kim, V. Maciulyte, J. Kleinjung, J.-S. Kim, D. Wells, L. Vallier, A. Bertero, J. M. A. Turner, and K. K. Niakan. 2017. Genome editing reveals a role for OCT4 in human embryogenesis. *Nature* 551(7674):67–73.

Fragouli, E., S. Alfarawati, K. Spath, D. Babariya, N. Tarozzi, A. Borini, and D. Wells. 2017. Analysis of implantation and ongoing pregnancy rates following the transfer of mosaic diploid-aneuploid blastocysts. *Human Genetics* 136(7):805–819.

Franasiak, J. M., E. J. Forman, K. H. Hong, M. D. Werner, K. M. Upham, N. R. Treff, and R. T. Scott Jr. 2014. The nature of aneuploidy with increasing age of the female partner: A review of 15,169 consecutive trophectoderm biopsies evaluated with comprehensive chromosomal screening. *Fertility and Sterility* 101(3):656–663.

Frum, T., M. A. Halbisen, C. Wang, H. Amiri, P. Robson, and A. Ralston. 2013. OCT4 cell-autonomously promotes primitive endoderm development in the mouse blastocyst. *Developmental Cell* 25(6):610–622.

Fukuta, M., Y. Nakai, K. Kirino, M. Nakagawa, K. Sekiguchi, S. Nagata, Y. Matsumoto, T. Yamamoto, K. Umeda, T. Heike, N. Okumura, N. Koizumi, T. Sato, T. Nakahata, M. Saito, T. Otsuka, S. Kinoshita, M. Ueno, M. Ikeya, and J. Toguchida. 2014. Derivation of mesenchymal stromal cells from pluripotent stem cells through a neural crest lineage using small molecule compounds with defined media. *PLOS ONE* 9(12):e112291.

Gao, X., D. Ruan, J. Wu, P. Liu, X. Gao, X. Chen, D. Ryan, J. Yang, L. Antunes, L. S. Campos, B. Fu, Y. Yong, F. Yang, S. A. Teichmann, P. Liu, M. Nowak-Imialek, D. Herrmann, S. Petkov, H. Niemann, M. Nowak-Imialek, D. Herrmann, S. Petkov, H. Niemann, D. Chen, J. Zhong, J. Zhu, S. Wang, Z. Shang, D. Chen, J. Zhong, J. Zhu, S. Wang, Z. Shang, D. Ruan, X. Wang, T. Nie, P. Li, D. Wu, D. Pei, L. Lai, A. C. H. Chen, Y. L. Lee, W. S. B. Yeung, M. A. Eckersley-Maslin, W. Reik, S. Ahmad, A. Ahmed, T. Kobayashi, A. Surani, G. Lan, X. Zou, S. G. Xue, L. Ge, Z. Liu, Y. Huang, D. Pei, Y. Zhang, L. Lu, S. J. Kimber, P. P. L. Tam, S. Petkov, J. Yang, and H. Niemann. 2019. Establishment of porcine and human expanded potential stem cells. *Nature Cell Biology* 21(6):687–699.

Gerami-Naini, B., O. V. Dovzhenko, M. Durning, F. H. Wegner, J. A. Thomson, and T. G. Golos. 2004. Trophoblast differentiation in embryoid bodies derived from human embryonic stem cells. *Endocrinology* 145:1517–1524.

Giakoumopoulos, M., and T. G. Golos. 2013. Embryonic stem cell-derived trophoblast differentiation: A comparative review of the biology, function, and signaling mechanisms. *Journal of Endocrinology.* 216(3):R33–R45.

Gleicher, N., A. Vidali, J. Braverman, V. A. Kushnir, D. H. Barad, C. Hudson, Y.-G. Wu, Q. Wang, L. Zhang, and D. F. Albertini. 2016. Accuracy of preimplantation genetic screening (PGS) is compromised by degree of mosaicism of human embryos. *Reproductive Biology and Endocrinology* 14(1):54.

Gomez, G. A., M. S. Prasad, N. Sandhu, P. B. Shelar, A. W. Leung, and M. I. García-Castro. 2019a. Human neural crest induction by temporal modulation of Wnt activation. *Developmental Biology* 449(2):99–106.

Gomez, G. A., M. S. Prasad, M. Wong, R. M. Charney, P. B. Shelar, N. Sandhu, J. O. S. Hackland, J. C. Hernandez, A. W. Leung, and M. I. García-Castro. 2019b. WNT/β-catenin modulates the axial identity of embryonic stem cell-derived human neural crest. *Development* 146(16):dev175604.

Graham, S. J. L., and M. Zernicka-Goetz. 2016. The acquisition of cell fate in mouse development: How do cells first become heterogeneous? *Current Topics in Developmental Biology* 117:671–695.

Graham, S. J., K. B. Wicher, A. Jedrusik, G. Guo, W. Herath, P. Robson, and M. Zernicka-Goetz. 2014. BMP signaling regulates the pre-implantation development of extra-embryonic cell lineages in the mouse embryo. *Nature Communications* 5(1):1–11.

Greco, E., M. G. Minasi, and F. Fiorentino. 2015. Healthy babies after intrauterine transfer of mosaic aneuploid blastocysts. *New England Journal of Medicine* 373(21):2089–2090.

Hackland, J. O. S., P. B. Shelar, N. Sandhu, M. S. Prasad, R. M. Charney, G. A. Gomez, T. J. R. Frith, and M. I. García-Castro. 2019. FGF modulates the axial identity of trunk hPSC-derived neural crest but not the cranial-trunk decision. *Stem Cell Reports* 12(5):920–933.

Haider, S., G. Meinhardt, L. Saleh, V. Kunihs, M. Gamperl, U. Kaindl, A. Ellinger, T. R. Burkard, C. Fiala, J. Pollheimer, S. Mendjan, P.A. Latos, and M. Knöfler. 2018. Self-renewing trophoblast organoids recapitulate the developmental program of the early human placenta. *Stem Cell Reports* 11(2):537–551.

Haller, M., Y. Yin, and L. Ma. 2019. Development and utilization of human decidualization reporter cell line uncovers new modulators of female fertility. *Proceedings of the National Academy of Sciences* 116(39):19541–19551.

Hardy, K., S. Spanos, D. Becker, P. Iannelli, R. M. L. Winston, and J. Stark. 2001. From cell death to embryo arrest: Mathematical models of human preimplantation embryo development. *Proceedings of the National Academy of Sciences* 98(4):1655–1660.

Harrison, S. E., B. Sozen, N. Christodoulou, C. Kyprianou, and M. Zernicka-Goetz. 2017. Assembly of embryonic and extraembryonic stem cells to mimic embryogenesis in vitro. *Science* 356(6334):eaal1810.

Heemskerk, I., K. Burt, M. Miller, S. Chhabra, M. C. Guerra, L. Liu, and A. Warmflash. 2019. Rapid changes in morphogen concentration control self-organized patterning in human embryonic stem cells. *eLife* 8:e40536.

Hertig, A. T., J. Rock, and E. C. Adams. 1956. A description of 34 human ova within the first 17 days of development. *American Journal of Anatomy* 98(3):435–493.

His, W. 1868. *Die erste Entwickelung des Hühnchens im Ei.* Leipzig, Germany: Vogel.

Hodgen, G. D., W. W. Tullner, J. L. Vaitukaitis, D. N. Ward, and G. T. Ross. 1974. Specific radioimmunoassay of chorionic gonadotropin during implantation in rhesus monkeys. *Journal of Clinical Endocrinology & Metabolism* 39(3):457–464.

Horii, M., Y. Li, A. K. Wakeland, D. P. Pizzo, K. K. Nelson, K. Sabatini, L. C. Laurent, Y. Liu, and M. M. Parast. 2016. Human pluripotent stem cells as a model of trophoblast differentiation in both normal development and disease. *Proceedings of the National Academy of Sciences* 113(27):E3882–E3891.

Horii, M., T. Bui, O. Touma, H. Y. Cho, and M. M. Parast. 2019. An improved two-step protocol for trophoblast differentiation of human pluripotent stem cells. *Current Protocols in Stem Cell Biology* 50(1):e96.

Hornak, M., D. Kubicek, P. Broz, P. Hulinska, K. Hanzalova, D. Griffin, M. Machatkova, and J. Rubes. 2016. Aneuploidy detection and mtdna quantification in bovine embryos with different cleavage onset using a next-generation sequencing-based protocol. *Cytogenetic and Genome Research* 150(1):60–67.

Huang, J., N. Zhao, X. Wang, J. Qiao, and P. Liu. 2015. Chromosomal characteristics at cleavage and blastocyst stages from the same embryos. *Journal of Assisted Reproduction and Genetics* 32(5):781–787.

Hyun, I., M. Munsie, M. F. Pera, N. C. Rivron, and J. Rossant. 2020. Toward guidelines for research on human embryo models formed from stem cells. *Stem Cell Reports* 14(2):169–174.

Irani, M., D. Reichman, A. Robles, A. Melnick, O. Davis, N. Zaninovic, K. Xu, and Z. Rosenwaks. 2017. Morphologic grading of euploid blastocysts influences implantation and ongoing pregnancy rates. *Fertility and Sterility* 107(3):664–670.

Jain, A., T. Ezashi, R. M. Roberts, and G. Tuteja. 2017. Deciphering transcriptional regulation in human embryonic stem cells specified towards a trophoblast fate. *Scientific Reports* 7(1):17257.

Johnson, D. S., C. Cinnioglu, R. Ross, A. Filby, G. Gemelos, M. Hill, A. Ryan, D. Smotrich, M. Rabinowitz, and M. J. Murray. 2010. Comprehensive analysis of karyotypic mosaicism between trophectoderm and inner cell mass. *Molecular Human Reproduction* 16(12):944–949.

Kalinka, A. T., and P. Tomancak. 2012. The evolution of early animal embryos: Conservation or divergence? *Trends in Ecology & Evolution* 27(7):385–393.

Kime, C., H. Kiyonari, S. Ohtsuka, E. Kohbayashi, M. Asahi, S. Yamanaka, M. Takahashi, and K. Tomoda. 2019. Induced 2C expression and implantation-competent blastocyst-like cysts from primed pluripotent stem cells. *Stem Cell Reports* 13(3):485–498.

Kobayashi, T., H. Zhang, W. W. C. Tang, N. Irie, S. Withey, D. Klisch, A. Sybirna, S. Dietmann, D. A. Contreras, R. Webb, C. Allegrucci, R. Alberio, and M. A. Surani. 2017. Principles of early human development and germ cell program from conserved model systems. *Nature* 546(7658):416–420.

Kojima, Y., K. Kaufman-Francis, J. B. Studdert, K. A. Steiner, M. D. Power, D. A. F. Loebel, V. Jones, A. Hor, G. de Alencastro, G. J. Logan, E. T. Teber, O. H. Tam, M. D. Stutz, I. E. Alexander, H. A. Pickett, and P. P. L. Tam. 2014. The transcriptional and functional properties of mouse epiblast stem cells resemble the anterior primitive streak. *Cell Stem Cell* 14(1):107–120.

Kojima, Y., K. Sasaki, S. Yokobayashi, Y. Sakai, T. Nakamura, Y. Yabuta, F. Nakaki, S. Nagaoka, K. Woltjen, and A. Hotta. 2017. Evolutionarily distinctive transcriptional and signaling programs drive human germ cell lineage specification from pluripotent stem cells. *Cell Stem Cell* 21(4):517–532.

Kolle, G., K. Krishnan, N. Cloonan, S. M. Grimmond, M. Ho, Z. Qi, H. S. Chy, I. Bertoncello, and A. L. Laslett. 2009. Identification of human embryonic stem cell surface markers by combined membrane-polysome translation state array analysis and immunotranscriptional profiling. *Stem Cells* 27(10):2446–2456.

Koot, Y. E. M., G. Teklenburg, M. S. Salker, J. J. Brosens, and N. S. Macklon. 2012. Molecular aspects of implantation failure. *Biochimica et Biophysica Acta* 1822(12):1943–1950.

Kunath, T., D. Arnaud, G. D. Uy, I. Okamoto, C. Chureau, Y. Yamanaka, E. Heard, R. L. Gardner, P. Avner, and J. Rossant. 2005. Imprinted X-inactivation in extra-embryonic endoderm cell lines from mouse blastocysts. *Development* 132(7):1649–1661.

Kurek, D., A. Neagu, M. Tastemel, N. Tüysüz, J. Lehmann, H. Werken, S. Philipsen, R. van der Linden, A. Maas, W. IJcken, M. Drukker, and D. Berge. 2015. Endogenous WNT signals mediate BMP-induced and spontaneous differentiation of epiblast stem cells and human embryonic stem cells. *Stem Cell Reports* 4(1):114–128.

Laslett, A. L., S. Grimmond, B. Gardiner, L. Stamp, A. Lin, S. M. Hawes, S. Wormald, D. Nikolic-Paterson, D. Haylock, and M. F. Pera. 2007. Transcriptional analysis of early lineage commitment in human embryonic stem cells. *BMC Developmental Biology* 7(1):1–18.

Lee, C. Q. E., L. Gardner, M. Turco, N. Zhao, M. J. Murray, N. Coleman, J. Rossant, M. Hemberger, and A. Moffett. 2016. What is trophoblast? A combination of criteria define human first-trimester trophoblast. *Stem Cell Reports* 6(2):257–272.

Lee, G., H. Kim, Y. Elkabetz, G. Al Shamy, G. Panagiotakos, T. Barberi, V. Tabar, and L. Studer. 2007a. Isolation and directed differentiation of neural crest stem cells derived from human embryonic stem cells. *Nature Biotechnology* 25(12):1468–1475.

Lee, Y., K. R. Kim, F. McKeon, A. Yang, T. K. Boyd, C. P. Crum, and M. M. Parast. 2007b. A unifying concept of trophoblastic differentiation and malignancy defined by biomarker expression. *Human Pathology* 38(7):1003–1013.

Leung, A. W., B. Murdoch, A. F. Salem, M. S. Prasad, G. A. Gomez, and M. I. García-Castro. 2016. Wnt/β-catenin signaling mediates human neural crest induction via a pre-neural border intermediate. *Development* 143(3):398–410.

Leung, A. W., F. López-Giráldez, C. Broton, K. Lin, M. S. Prasad, J. C. Hernández, A. Z. Xiao, and M. I. García-Castro. 2019. Pre-border gene Ffoxb1 regulates the differentiation timing and autonomic neuronal potential of human neural crest cells. *bioRxiv* 646026.

Li, R., C. Zhong, Y. Yu, H. Liu, M. Sakurai, L. Yu, Z. Min, L. Shi, Y. Wei, Y. Takahashi, H.-K. Liao, J. Qiao, H. Deng, E. Nuòez-Delicado, C. Rodriguez Esteban, J. Wu, and J. C. Izpisua Belmonte. 2019. Generation of blastocyst-like structures from mouse embryonic and adult cell cultures. *Cell* 179(3):687–702.

Li, Y., M. Moretto-Zita, F. Soncin, A. Wakeland, L. Wolfe, S. Leon-Garcia, R. Pandian, D. Pizzo, L. Cui, K. Nazor, J. F. Loring, C. P. Crum, L. C. Laurent, and M. M. Parast. 2013. BMP4-directed trophoblast differentiation of human embryonic stem cells is mediated through a Np63 + cytotrophoblast stem cell state. *Development* 140(19):3965–3976.

Lightfoot, D. A., A. Kouznetsova, E. Mahdy, J. Wilbertz, and C. Höög. 2006. The fate of mosaic aneuploid embryos during mouse development. *Developmental Biology* 289(2):384–394.

Linneberg-Agerholm, M., Y. F. Wong, J. A. Romero Herrera, R. S. Monteiro, K. G. V. Anderson, and J. M. Brickman. 2019. Naive human pluripotent stem cells respond to Wnt, Nodal and LIF signalling to produce expandable naive extra-embryonic endoderm. *Development (Cambridge, England)* 146(24):dev180620.

Liu, S., M. Kwon, M. Mannino, N. Yang, F. Renda, A. Khodjakov, and D. Pellman. 2018. Nuclear envelope assembly defects link mitotic errors to chromothripsis. *Nature* 561(7724):551–555.

Luckett, P. 1976. Cladistic relationships among primate higher categories: Evidence of the fetal membranes and placenta. *Folia Primatologica* 25(4):245–276.

Ma, H., J. Zhai, H. Wan, X. Jiang, X. Wang, L. Wang, Y. Xiang, X. He, Z.-A. Zhao, B. Zhao, P. Zheng, L. Li, and H. Wang. 2019. In vitro culture of cynomolgus monkey embryos beyond early gastrulation. *Science* 366(6467):eaax7890.

Macaulay, I. C., W. Haerty, P. Kumar, Y. I. Li, T. X. Hu, M. J. Teng, M. Goolam, N. Saurat, P. Coupland, and L. M. Shirley. 2015. G&T-seq: Parallel sequencing of single-cell genomes and transcriptomes. *Nature Methods* 12(6):519–522.

Macfarlan, T. S., W. D. Gifford, S. Driscoll, K. Lettieri, H. M. Rowe, D. Bonanomi, A. Firth, O. Singer, D. Trono, and S. L. Pfaff. 2012. Embryonic stem cell potency fluctuates with endogenous retrovirus activity. *Nature* 487(7405):57–63.

Macklon, N. S., J. P. M. Geraedts, and B. C. J. M. Fauser. 2002. Conception to ongoing pregnancy: The black box of early pregnancy loss. *Human Reproduction* 8(4):333–343.

Marshall, A. M. 1879. The morphology of the vertebrate olfactory organ. *Journal of Cell Science* 19(75):300–340.

Martin, G. R. 1981. Isolation of a pluripotent cell line from early mouse embryos cultured in medium conditioned by teratocarcinoma stem cells. *Proceedings of the National Academy of Sciences* 78(12):7634–7638.

Martyn, I., T. Y. Kanno, A. Ruzo, E. D. Siggia, and A. H. Brivanlou. 2018. Self-organization of a human organizer by combined Wnt and Nodal signalling. *Nature* 558:132–135.

Martyn, I., A. H. Brivanlou, and E. D. Siggia. 2019. A wave of Wnt signaling balanced by secreted inhibitors controls primitive streak formation in micropattern colonies of human embryonic stem cells. *Development* 146(6):dev172791.

Massey, J., Y. Liu, O. Alvarenga, T. Saez, M. Schmerer, and A. Warmflash. 2019. Synergy with TGFβ ligands switches WNT pathway dynamics from transient to sustained during human pluripotent cell differentiation. *Proceedings of the National Academy of Sciences* 116(11):4989–4998.

Maurer, M., T. Ebner, M. Puchner, R. Bernhard Mayer, O. Shebl, P. Oppelt, and H. C. Duba. 2015. Chromosomal aneuploidies and early embryonic developmental arrest. *International Journal of Fertility and Sterility* 9(3):346–353.

McCoy, R. C. 2017. Mosaicism in preimplantation human embryos: When chromosomal abnormalities are the norm. *Trends in Genetics* 33(7):448–463.

McCoy, R. C., Z. P. Demko, A. Ryan, M. Banjevic, M. Hill, S. Sigurjonsson, M. Rabinowitz, and D. A. Petrov. 2015. Evidence of selection against complex mitotic-origin aneuploidy during preimplantation development. *PLOS Genetics* 11(10):e1005601.

Menendez, L., T. A. Yatskievych, P. B. Antin, and S. Dalton. 2011. Wnt signaling and a Smad pathway blockade direct the differentiation of human pluripotent stem cells to multipotent neural crest cells. *Proceedings of the National Academy of Sciences* 108(48):19240–19245.

Mica, Y., G. Lee, S. M. Chambers, M. J. Tomishima, and L. Studer. 2013. Modeling neural crest induction, melanocyte specification, and disease-related pigmentation defects in hESCs and patient-specific iPSCs. *Cell Reports* 3(4):1140–1152.

Morris, S. A., S. Grewal, F. Barrios, S. N. Patankar, B. Strauss, L. Buttery, M. Alexander, K. M. Shakesheff, and M. Zernicka-Goetz. 2012. Dynamics of anterior–posterior axis formation in the developing mouse embryo. *Nature Communications* 3(1):1–10.

Munné, S., J. Grifo, J. Cohen, and H. U. Weier. 1994. Chromosome abnormalities in human arrested preimplantation embryos: A multiple-probe FISH study. *American Journal of Human Genetics* 55(1):150–159.

Murdoch, B., C. DelConte, and M. I. García-Castro. 2010. Embryonic Pax7-expressing progenitors contribute multiple cell types to the postnatal olfactory epithelium. *Journal of Neuroscience* 30(28):9523–9532.

Murdoch, B., C. DelConte, and M. I. García-Castro. 2012. Pax7 lineage contributions to the mammalian neural crest. *PLOS ONE* 7(7):e41089.

Nakamura, T., I. Okamoto, K. Sasaki, Y. Yabuta, C. Iwatani, H. Tsuchiya, Y. Seita, S. Nakamura, T. Yamamoto, and M. Saitou. 2016. A developmental coordinate of pluripotency among mice, monkeys and humans. *Nature* 537(7618):57–62.

Nazem, T. G., L. Sekhon, J. A. Lee, J. Overbey, S. Pan, M. Duke, C. Briton-Jones, M. Whitehouse, A. B. Copperman, and D. E. Stein. 2019. The correlation between morphology and implantation of euploid human blastocysts. *Reproduction and Biomedicine Online* 38(2):169–176.

Nemashkalo, A., A. Ruzo, I. Heemskerk, and A. Warmflash. 2017. Morphogen and community effects determine cell fates in response to BMP4 signaling in human embryonic stem cells. *Development* 144(17):3042–3053.

Niakan, K. K., and K. Eggan. 2013. Analysis of human embryos from zygote to blastocyst reveals distinct gene expression patterns relative to the mouse. *Developmental Biology* 375(1):54–64.

Nishioka, N., K.-I. Inoue, K. Adachi, H. Kiyonari, M. Ota, A. Ralston, N. Yabuta, S. Hirahara, R. O. Stephenson, N. Ogonuki, R. Makita, H. Kurihara, E. M. Morin-Kensicki, H. Nojima, J. Rossant, K. Nakao, H. Niwa, and H. Sasaki. 2009. The Hippo signaling pathway components Lats and Yap pattern Tead4 activity to distinguish mouse trophectoderm from inner cell mass. *Developmental cell* 16(3):398–410.

Niu, Y., N. Sun, C. Li, Y. Lei, Z. Huang, J. Wu, C. Si, X. Dai, C. Liu, J. Wei, L. Liu, S. Feng, Y. Kang, W. Si, H. Wang, E. Zhang, L. Zhao, Z. Li, X. Luo, G. Cui, G. Peng, J. C. Izpis'a Belmonte, W. Ji, and T. Tan. 2019. Dissecting primate early post-implantation development using long-term in vitro embryo culture. *Science* 366(6467):eaaw5754.

Okae, H., H. Toh, T. Sato, H. Hiura, S. Takahashi, K. Shirane, Y. Kabayama, M. Suyama, H. Sasaki, and T. Arima. 2018. Derivation of human trophoblast stem cells. *Cell Stem Cell* 22(1):50–63.

Pereda, J., and H. B. Croxatto. 1978. Ultrastructure of a seven-cell human embryo. *Biology of Reproduction* 18(3):481–489.

Petropoulos, S., D. Edsgärd, B. R. Reinius, Q. Deng, S. P. Panula, S. Codeluppi, A. Plaza Reyes, S. Linnarsson, R. Sandberg, and F. Lanner. 2016. Single-cell RNA-seq reveals lineage and X chromosome dynamics in human preimplantation embryos. *Cell* 165(4):1012–1026.

Pomp, O., I. Brokhman, I. Ben-Dor, B. Reubinoff, and R. S. Goldstein. 2005. Generation of peripheral sensory and sympathetic neurons and neural crest cells from human embryonic stem cells. *Stem Cells* 23(7):923–930.

Posfai, E., S. Petropoulos, F. R. O. de Barros, J. P. Schell, I. Jurisica, R. Sandberg, F. Lanner, and J. Rossant. 2017. Position- and Hippo signaling-dependent plasticity during lineage segregation in the early mouse embryo. *eLife* 6:e22906.

Ramanujam, R., T. Y. F. Low, Y. W. Lim, and F. Motegi. 2017. Forceful patterning in mouse preimplantation embryos. *YSCDB Seminars in Cell and Developmental Biology* 71:129–136.

Rambags, B. P., P. J. Krijtenburg, H. F. Drie, G. Lazzari, C. Galli, P. L. Pearson, B. Colenbrander, and T. A. Stout. 2005. Numerical chromosomal abnormalities in equine embryos produced in vivo and in vitro. *Molecular Reproduction and Development* 72(1):77–87.

Rivron, N., M. Pera, J. Rossant, A. M. Arias, M. Zernicka-Goetz, J. Fu, S. van den Brink, A. Bredenoord, W. Dondorp, and G. de Wert. 2018a. Debate ethics of embryo models from stem cells. *Nature* 564(7735):183–185.

Rivron, N. C., J. Frias-Aldeguer, E. J. Vrij, R. K. Truckenmuller, C. A. van Blitterswijk, N. C. Rivron, J. Frias-Aldeguer, J. C. Boisset, J. Korving, J. Vivie, A. van Oudenaarden, N. Geijsen, J. Vivie, and N. Geijsen. 2018b. Blastocyst-like structures generated solely from stem cells. *Nature* 557(7703):106–111.

Roberts, R. M., T. Ezashi, M. A. Sheridan, R. M. Roberts, M. A. Sheridan, R. M. Roberts, T. Ezashi, and Y. Yang. 2018. Specification of trophoblast from embryonic stem cells exposed to BMP4. *Biology of Reproduction* 99(1):212–224.

Rossant, J., and P. P. L. Tam. 2017. New insights into early human development: Lessons for stem cell derivation and differentiation. *Cell Stem Cell* 20(1):18–28.

Ruzo, A., G. F. Croft, J. J. Metzger, S. Galgoczi, L. J. Gerber, C. Pellegrini, H. Wang, Jr., M. Fenner, S. Tse, A. Marks, C. Nchako, and A. H. Brivanlou. 2018. Chromosomal instability during neurogenesis in Huntington's disease. *Development* 145(2):dev156844.

Sasaki, K., T. Nakamura, I. Okamoto, Y. Yabuta, C. Iwatani, H. Tsuchiya, Y. Seita, S. Nakamura, N. Shiraki, T. Takakuwa, T. Yamamoto, and M. Saitou. 2016. The germ cell fate of cynomolgus monkeys is specified in the nascent amnion. *Developmental Cell* 39(2):169–185.

Seguin, C. A., J. S. Draper, A. Nagy, and J. Rossant. 2008. Establishment of endoderm progenitors by SOX transcription factor expression in human embryonic stem cells. *Cell Stem Cell* 3(2):182–195.

Shahbazi, M. N., A. Jedrusik, S. Vuoristo, G. Recher, A. Hupalowska, V. Bolton, N. M. Fogarty, A. Campbell, L. G. Devito, and D. Ilic. 2016. Self-organization of the human embryo in the absence of maternal tissues. *Nature Cell Biology* 18(6):700–708.

Shahbazi, M. N., A. Scialdone, N. Skorupska, A. Weberling, G. Recher, M. Zhu, A. Jedrusik, L. G. Devito, L. Noli, and I. C. Macaulay. 2017. Pluripotent state transitions coordinate morphogenesis in mouse and human embryos. *Nature* 552(7684):239–243.

Shahbazi, M. N., and M. Zernicka-Goetz. 2018. Deconstructing and reconstructing the mouse and human early embryo. *Nature Cell Biology* 20(8):878–887.

Shao, Y., K. Taniguchi, K. Gurdziel, R. F. Townshend, X. Xue, K. M. Yong, J. Sang, J. R. Spence, D. L. Gumucio, and J. Fu. 2017a. Self-organized amniogenesis by human pluripotent stem cells in a biomimetic implantation-like niche. *Nature Materials* 16(4):419–425.

Shao, Y., K. Taniguchi, R. F. Townshend, T. Miki, D. L. Gumucio, and J. Fu. 2017b. A pluripotent stem cell-based model for post-implantation human amniotic sac development. *Nature Communications* 8(1):208.

Sheridan, M. A., V. Balaraman, D. J. Schust, T. Ezashi, R. M. Roberts, and A. W. E. Franz. 2018. African and Asian strains of Zika virus differ in their ability to infect and lyse primitive human placental trophoblast. *PLOS ONE* 13(7).

Sheridan, M. A., Y. Yang, A. Jain, A. S. Lyons, P. Yang, S. R. Brahmasani, A. Dai, Y. Tian, M. R. Ellersieck, G. Tuteja, D. J. Schust, L. C. Schulz, T. Ezashi, and R. M. Roberts. 2019. Early onset preeclampsia in a model for human placental trophoblast. *Proceedings of the National Academy of Sciences* 116(10):4336–4345.

Silver, L. M. 1995. *Mouse genetics: Concepts and applications*. New York: Oxford University Press.

Simunovic, M., J. J. Metzger, F. Etoc, A. Yoney, A. Ruzo, I. Martyn, G. Croft, D. S. You, A. H. Brivanlou, and E. D. Siggia. 2019. A 3D model of a human epiblast reveals BMP4-driven symmetry breaking. *Nature Cell Biology* 21(7):900–910.

Soncin, F., M. Khater, C. To, D. Pizzo, O. Farah, A. Wakeland, K. Arul Nambi Rajan, K. K. Nelson, C. W. Chang, M. Moretto-Zita, D. R. Natale, L. C. Laurent, and M. M. Parast. 2018. Comparative analysis of mouse and human placentae across gestation reveals species-specific regulators of placental development. *Development* 145(2):dev156273.

Sozen, B., G. Amadei, A. Cox, R. Wang, Ellen, S. Czukiewska, L. Chappell, T. Voet, G. Michel, N. Jing, D. M. Glover, and M. Zernicka-Goetz. 2018. Self-assembly of embryonic and two extra-embryonic stem cell types into gastrulating embryo-like structures. *Nature Cell Biology* 20(8):979–989.

Sozen, B., A. L. Cox, J. De Jonghe, M. Bao, F. Hollfelder, D. M. Glover, and M. Zernicka-Goetz. 2019. Self-organization of mouse stem cells into an extended potential blastoid. *Developmental Cell* 51(6):698–712.

Steptoe, P. C., and R. G. Edwards. 1978. Birth after the reimplantation of a human embryo. *Lancet* 2(8085):366.

Stevens, V. C. 1997. Some reproductive studies in the baboon. *Human Reproduction Update* 3(6):533–540.

Stirparo, G. G., T. Boroviak, G. Guo, J. Nichols, A. Smith, and P. Bertone. 2018. Integrated analysis of single-cell embryo data yields a unified transcriptome signature for the human pre-implantation epiblast. *Development* 145(3):dev158501.

Tanaka, S., T. Kunath, A. K. Hadjantonakis, A. Nagy, and J. Rossant. 1998. Promotion of trophoblast stem cell proliferation by FGF4. *Science* 282(5396):2072–2075.

Theunissen, T. W., and R. Jaenisch. 2017. Mechanisms of gene regulation in human embryos and pluripotent stem cells. *Development* 144(24):4496–4509.

Thomson, J. A., J. Kalishman, T. G. Golos, M. Durning, C. P. Harris, R. A. Becker, and J. P. Hearn. 1995. Isolation of a primate embryonic stem cell line. *Proceedings of the National Academy of Sciences* 92(17):7844–7848.

Thomson, J. A., J. Itskovitz-Eldor, S. S. Shapiro, M. A. Waknitz, J. J. Swiergiel, V. S. Marshall, and J. M. Jones. 1998. Embryonic stem cell lines derived from human blastocysts. *Science* 282(5391):1145–1147.

Treff, N. R., X. Tao, H. Garnsey, C. Bohrer, J. Landis, D. Taylor, R. T. Scott, N. R. Treff, J. Landis, D. Taylor, R. T. Scott, R. L. Krisher, E. Silva, T. K. Woodruff, and F. E. Duncan. 2016. Next generation sequencing-based comprehensive chromosome screening in mouse polar bodies, oocytes, and embryos. *Biology of Reproduction* 94(4):76.

Tšuiko, O., M. Catteeuw, M. Zamani Esteki, A. Destouni, O. Bogado Pascottini, U. Besenfelder, V. Havlicek, K. Smits, A. Kurg, A. Salumets, T. D'Hooghe, T. Voet, A. Van Soom, and J. Robert Vermeesch. 2017. Genome stability of bovine in vivo-conceived cleavage-stage embryos is higher compared to in vitro-produced embryos. *Human Reproduction* 32(11):2348–2357.

Turco, M. Y., and A. Moffett. 2019. Development of the human placenta. *Development* 146(22):dev163428.

Vanneste, E., T. Voet, C. Melotte, S. Debrock, K. Sermon, C. Staessen, I. Liebaers, J. P. Fryns, T. Dhooghe, and J. R. Vermeesch. 2009a. What next for preimplantation genetic screening? High mitotic chromosome instability rate provides the biological basis for the low success rate. *Human Reproduction* 24(11):2679–2682.

Vanneste, E., T. Voet, C. Le Caignec, M. Ampe, P. Konings, C. Melotte, S. Debrock, M. Amyere, M. Vikkula, F. Schuit, J. P. Fryns, G. Verbeke, T. D'Hooghe, Y. Moreau, and J. R. Vermeesch. 2009b. Chromosome instability is common in human cleavage-stage embryos. *Nature Medicine* 15(5):577–583.

Vazquez-Diez, C., J. Haverfield, G. FitzHarris, K. Yamagata, S. Trivedi, and G. FitzHarris. 2016. Micronucleus formation causes perpetual unilateral chromosome inheritance in mouse embryos. *Proceedings of the National Academy of Sciences* 113(3):626–631.

Wamaitha, S. E., K. J. Grybel, G. Alanis-Lobato, C. Gerri, S. Ogushi, A. McCarthy, S. K. Mahadevaiah, L. Healy, R. A. Lea, M. Molina-Arcas, L. G. Devito, K. Elder, P. Snell, L. Christie, J. Downward, J. M. A. Turner, and K. K. Niakan. 2020. IGF1-mediated human embryonic stem cell self-renewal recapitulates the embryonic niche. *Nature Communications* 11(1).

Warmflash, A., B. Sorre, F. Etoc, E. D. Siggia, A. Warmflash, B. Sorre, F. Etoc, and A. H. Brivanlou. 2014. A method to recapitulate early embryonic spatial patterning in human embryonic stem cells. *Nature Methods* 11(8):847–854.

West, R., H. Ming, D. Logsdon, J. Sun, S. Rajput, R. Kile, W. Schoolcraft, R. Roberts, R. Krisher, Z. Jiang, and Y. Yuan. 2019. Dynamics of trophoblast differentiation in peri-implantation-stage human embryos. *Proceedings of the National Academy of Sciences* 116(45):22635–22644.

Wigger, M., K. Kisielewska, K. Filimonow, B. Plusa, M. Maleszewski, and A. Suwinska. 2017. Plasticity of the inner cell mass in mouse blastocyst is restricted by the activity of FGF/MAPK pathway. *Scientific Reports* 7(1):15136.

Wilcox, A. J., C. R. Weinberg, J. F. O'Connor, D. D. Baird, J. P. Schlatterer, R. E. Canfield, E. G. Armstrong, and B. C. Nisula. 1988. Incidence of early loss of pregnancy. *New England Journal of Medicine* 319(4):189–194.

Wilson, S. I., A. Rydstrom, T. Trimborn, K. Willert, R. Nusse, T. M. Jessell, and T. Edlund. 2001. The status of Wnt signalling regulates neural and epidermal fates in the chick embryo. *Nature* 411(6835):325–330.

Xu, R. H., X. Chen, D. S. Li, R. Li, G. C. Addicks, C. Glennon, T. P. Zwaka, and J. A. Thomson. 2002. BMP4 initiates human embryonic stem cell differentiation to trophoblast. *Nature Biotechnology* 20(12):1261–1264.

Yabe, S., A. P. Alexenko, M. Amita, Y. Yang, D. J. Schust, Y. Sadovsky, T. Ezashi, and R. M. Roberts. 2016. Comparison of syncytiotrophoblast generated from human embryonic stem cells and from term placentas. *Proceedings of the National Academy of Sciences* 113(19):E2598–E2607.

Yamaguchi, Y., and S. Yamada. 2018. The Kyoto Collection of Human Embryos and Fetuses: History and recent advancements in modern methods. *Cells Tissues Organs* 205(5–6):314–319.

Yamanaka, Y., F. Lanner, and J. Rossant. 2010. FGF signal-dependent segregation of primitive endoderm and epiblast in the mouse blastocyst. *Development* 137(5):715–724.

Yang, Y., K. Adachi, M. A. Sheridan, A. P. Alexenko, D. J. Schust, L. C. Schulz, T. Ezashi, and R. M. Roberts. 2015. Heightened potency of human pluripotent stem cell lines created by transient BMP4 exposure. *Proceedings of the National Academy of Sciences* 112(18):E2337–E2346.

Yang, J., D. J. Ryan, W. Wang, J. C. H. Tsang, X. Gao, L. Antunes, Y. Yu, Z. Zhu, J. Wang, A. A. Kolodziejczyk, L. S. Campos, C. Wang, F. Yang, B. Fu, M. Woods, X. Chen, J. Bussell, J. White, R. Ramirez-Solis, W. Reik, S. A. Teichmann, L. Lu, P. Liu, G. Lan, X. Zou, H. Masaki, H. Nakauchi, A. A. Kolodziejczyk, S. A. Teichmann, Z. Zhong, M. A. Eckersley-Maslin, W. Reik, Y. Tanaka, A. C. Wilkinson, B. Gottgens, Y. Tanaka, A. C. Wilkinson, B. Gottgens, Y. Tanaka, P. P. L. Tam, P. P. L. Tam, H. Nakauchi, and L. Lu. 2017a. Establishment of mouse expanded potential stem cells. *Nature* 550(7676):393–397.

Yang, Y., B. Liu, J. Xu, J. Wang, J. Wu, C. Shi, Y. Xu, J. Dong, C. Wang, W. Lai, J. Zhu, L. Xiong, D. Zhu, X. Li, W. Yang, T. Yamauchi, A. Sugawara, Z. Li, F. Sun, X. Li, C. Li, A. He, Y. Du, T. Wang, C. Zhao, H. Li, X. Chi, H. Zhang, Y. Liu, C. Li, S. Duo, M. Yin, H. Shen, J. C. I. Belmonte, and H. Deng. 2017b. Derivation of pluripotent stem cells with in vivo embryonic and extraembryonic potency. *Cell* 169(2):243–257.

Ying, Q.-L., J. Wray, J. Nichols, L. Batlle-Morera, B. Doble, J. Woodgett, P. Cohen, and A. Smith. 2008. The ground state of embryonic stem cell self-renewal. *Nature* 453(7194):519–523.

Yoney, A., F. Etoc, A. Ruzo, J. J. Metzger, I. Martyn, S. Li, A. H. Brivanlou, A. Yoney, F. Etoc, J. J. Metzger, I. Martyn, C. Kirst, E. D. Siggia, and T. Carroll. 2018. Wnt signaling memory is required for activin to function as a morphogen in human gastruloids. *eLife* 7:e38279.

Zhang, C.-Z., A. Spektor, H. Cornils, J. M. Francis, E. K. Jackson, S. Liu, M. Meyerson, and D. Pellman. 2015. Chromothripsis from DNA damage in micronuclei. *Nature* 522(7555):179–184.

Zheng, Y., X. Xue, Y. Shao, S. Wang, S. N. Esfahani, Z. Li, J. M. Muncie, J. N. Lakins, V. M. Weaver, D. L. Gumucio, and J. Fu. 2019. Controlled modelling of human epiblast and amnion development using stem cells. *Nature* 573(7774):421–425.

Zhou, F., R. Wang, P. Yuan, Y. Ren, Y. Mao, R. Li, Y. Lian, J. Li, L. Wen, L. Yan, J. Qiao, F. Tang, F. Zhou, R. Wang, Y. Mao, L. Wen, L. Yan, J. Qiao, F. Tang, P. Yuan, Y. Ren, R. Li, Y. Lian, J. Li, L. Yan, J. Qiao, F. Tang, L. Yan, J. Qiao, J. Qiao, F. Tang, J. Qiao, and F. Tang. 2019. Reconstituting the transcriptome and DNA methylome landscapes of human implantation. *Nature* 572(7771):660–664.

Zinaman, M. J., E. D. Clegg, C. C. Brown, J. O'Connor, and S. G. Selevan. 1996. Estimates of human fertility and pregnancy loss. *Fertility and Sterility* 65(3):503–509.

Appendix A

Workshop Agenda

Keck Center of the National Academies
Room 100
500 Fifth Street, NW
Washington, DC 20001

8:30 a.m. **Opening Remarks and Charge to Workshop Speakers and Participants**

MARTIN PERA
Professor
The Jackson Laboratory

8:45 a.m. **Opening Keynote Lecture**
Unique Aspects of Human Embryology and Opportunities and Challenges with Stem Cell–Based Embryo Models

JANET ROSSANT
Senior Scientist, Developmental and Stem Cell Biology
The Hospital for Sick Children

9:05 a.m. **Clarifying Questions from Workshop Participants**

SESSION I: MAMMALIAN EMBRYO RESEARCH AND PLURIPOTENT STEM CELLS

SESSION OBJECTIVE:

- Explore the characteristics of mammalian embryo model systems and the potential benefits and limitations to using these models for studying human embryonic development.

Session Moderator: Renee Reijo Pera, California Polytechnic State University

9:20 a.m. KATHY NIAKAN
Group Leader
Francis Crick Institute

9:35 a.m. MAGDALENA ZERNICKA-GOETZ
Professor of Mammalian Development and Stem Cell Biology
University of Cambridge
Bren Professor of Biology and Biological Engineering
California Institute of Technology

9:50 a.m. HEIDI COOK-ANDERSEN
Assistant Professor, Reproductive Medicine
University of California, San Diego

10:05 a.m. **Panel Discussion with Speakers and Workshop Participants**

10:35 a.m. **Break**

SESSION II: EXAMINING THE DEVELOPMENT OF EXTRAEMBRYONIC LINEAGES

SESSION OBJECTIVES:

- Explore the current state of the science about human extraembryonic lineages and how they are defined and characterized.
- Examine the impact of extraembryonic lineages on human embryo model systems.

Session Moderator: Amander Clark, University of California, Los Angeles

10:50 a.m. R. Michael Roberts
Chancellor's Professor, Animal Sciences and Biochemistry
University of Missouri

11:05 a.m. Mana Parast
Professor in Residence, Pathology
University of California, San Diego

11:20 a.m. Paul Robson
Associate Professor and Director, Single Cell Biology
The Jackson Laboratory

11:35 a.m. **Panel Discussion with Speakers and Workshop Participants**

12:05 p.m. **Break for Lunch**

SESSION III: STEM CELL–BASED MODELS OF HUMAN EMBRYOS

SESSION OBJECTIVES:

- Learn about the latest scientific and technical developments with models of human embryos and the direction for future research and applications of this work.
- Examine the fidelity of human embryo model systems to bona fide human embryos and explore methods for validation of the model systems.

Session Moderator: Arnold Kriegstein, University of California, San Francisco

1:10 p.m. Ali Brivanlou
Robert and Harriet Heilbrunn Professor
The Rockefeller University

1:25 p.m. Aryeh Warmflash
Principal Investigator
Assistant Professor, Department of Biosciences
Rice University

1:40 p.m. Nicolas Rivron
Group Leader, Institute of Molecular Biotechnology
Austrian Academy of Sciences

1:55 p.m. JIANPING FU
Associate Professor, Biomedical and Mechanical Engineering
Associate Professor, Cell and Developmental Biology
University of Michigan

2:10 p.m. **Panel Discussion with Speakers and Workshop Participants**

2:40 p.m. **Break**

SESSION IV: COMPARATIVE EMBRYONIC DEVELOPMENT ACROSS SPECIES

SESSION OBJECTIVES:

- Understand the similarities and differences between nonhuman embryos, embryo models (e.g., chimeras), and human embryos.
- Identify scientific questions that may necessitate the study of human embryos.

Session Moderator: Jianping Fu, University of Michigan

2:55 p.m. SHAWN CHAVEZ
Assistant Professor
Division of Reproductive and Developmental Sciences
Oregon Health & Science University

3:10 p.m. TED GOLOS
Professor and Chair
Department of Comparative Biosciences
University of Wisconsin

3:25 p.m. MARTÍN GARCÍA CASTRO
Associate Professor, Biomedical Sciences
Univerity of California, Riverside

3:40 p.m. JUN WU
Assistant Professor, Molecular Biology
University of Texas Southwestern Medical Center

3:55 p.m. **Panel Discussion with Speakers and Workshop Participants**

SESSION V: FUTURE OPPORTUNITIES AND CHALLENGES WITH MAMMALIAN EMBRYO MODEL SYSTEMS

SESSION OBJECTIVE:

- Summarize the lessons learned and topics discussed throughout the workshop, and address the key questions shown below.

Key Questions:

- What did we hear today that was new and could be moved forward to help advance the field?
- What was not discussed today that you think is important and key to the development of human embryo model systems?
- What level of fidelity exists between human embryo model systems and bona fide human embryos?

Session Moderator: Nicolas Rivron, Austrian Academy of Sciences

4:25 p.m. **Final Panel Discussion**

Ali Brivanlou
Jianping Fu
Kathy Niakan
Mana Parast

4:55 p.m. **Closing Keynote**

Martin Pera
Professor
The Jackson Laboratory

5:15 p.m. **Clarifying Questions from Workshop Participants**

5:25 p.m. **Final Remarks**

Janet Rossant
Senior Scientist, Developmental and Stem Cell Biology
The Hospital for Sick Children

5:30 p.m. **Adjourn**

Appendix B

Speaker Biographical Sketches

Richard Behringer, M.D., is a professor in the Department of Genetics and the Ben F. Love Chair for Cancer Research at The University of Texas MD Anderson Cancer Center in Houston, Texas. Dr. Behringer's research focuses on mammalian developmental genetics, including organogenesis, stem cells, and evolution. Dr. Behringer also conducts field studies on Kangaroo Island in Australia and on the Caribbean island of Trinidad. Previously, he was the director of the Molecular Embryology of the Mouse course at the Cold Spring Harbor Laboratory and the director of the Embryology course at the Marine Biological Laboratory in Woods Hole, Massachusetts. He is one of the editors of the 3rd and 4th editions of *Manipulating the Mouse Embryo: A Laboratory Manual* and the co-author with Dr. Virginia Papaioannou of *Mouse Phenotypes: A Handbook of Mutation Analysis*, both published by CSHL Press. Through social media (Twitter @rrbehringer), he is an advocate for developmental biology, genetics, and reproductive biology.

Ali Brivanlou, Ph.D., is the Robert and Harriet Heilbrunn Professor of Stem Cell Biology and Molecular Embryology at The Rockefeller University. Dr. Brivanlou received his doctoral degree in 1990 from the University of California, Berkeley, after receiving his M.S. in biochemistry from the Université des Sciences et Techniques du Languedoc. He joined The Rockefeller University in 1994 as an assistant professor after postdoctoral work in Douglas Melton's lab at Harvard University. Among his many awards are the Irma T. Hirschl/Monique Weill-Caulier Trusts Career Scientist Award, the Searle Scholar Award, the James A. Shannon Director's

Award from the National Institutes of Health, and the Presidential Early Career Award for Scientists and Engineers. Dr. Brivanlou also held research positions at International Genetic Engineering Inc. and the Molecular Biology Institute at the University of California, Los Angeles. Dr. Brivanlou has received more than 20 research funding awards and grants and is the recipient of, among numerous other honors, The Rockefeller University Teaching Award, the John Merck Award, the Presidential Early Career Award for Scientists and Engineers, and the Wilson S. Stone Memorial Award. He is currently a board member of the Research Foundation to Cure Aids, a member of the Scientific Advisory Council Pershing Square Sohn Cancer Research Alliance, a member of the Postdoctoral Awards Review Committee at The Rockefeller University, and the director of the Tri-Institutional (Memorial Sloan Kettering, Cornell Medical School, and The Rockefeller University) Human Embryonic Stem Cell Derivation Unit as well as the chair of its steering committee, among many other leadership positions at stem cell–focused initiatives.

Shawn L. Chavez, Ph.D., is an assistant professor in the Division of Reproductive and Developmental Sciences at the Oregon National Primate Research Center (ONPRC) as well as in the Department of Obstetrics and Gynecology and the Department of Physiology and Pharmacology at Oregon Health & Science University (OHSU), where she has been a faculty member since September 2013. Dr. Chavez obtained her Ph.D. in molecular, cellular, and developmental biology from Yale University and her B.S. in biological sciences from the University of California, Santa Barbara. She completed her postdoctoral training at the University of California, San Francisco, and at Stanford University. Her research interests focus on the use of real-time imaging and low-input next-generation sequencing to investigate the genetic, epigenetic, and chromosomal requirements of early embryogenesis and placentation in nonhuman primates and other mammals. In particular, her laboratory aims to determine how whole chromosomal abnormalities (aneuploidy) and sub-chromosomal instability may arise or be resolved during pre-implantation development. She is also actively examining the molecular and cellular connections between the formation of the placental-derived trophectoderm layer in embryos and subsequent placentation in normal pregnancies versus those complicated by preterm labor. Collectively, the goals of this research are to enhance our understanding of normal gametogenesis, embryogenesis, and placentation across different mammalian species, while improving in vitro fertilization outcomes for infertile couples and preventing embryo or fetal loss during pregnancy.

Amander Clark, Ph.D., is a professor in and the chair of the Department of Molecular Cell and Developmental Biology, University of California, Los Angeles (UCLA). She is a key member of the UCLA Eli & Edythe Broad Center of Regenerative Medicine and Stem Cell Research and an executive board member of the International Society for Stem Cell Research. As an independent principal investigator, Dr. Clark's research is focused on germline development, epigenetic reprogramming, and in vitro gametogenesis using pluripotent stem cells.

Heidi Cook-Andersen, M.D., Ph.D., is an assistant professor at the University of California, San Diego, with appointments in both the Department of Obstetrics, Gynecology, and Reproductive Sciences and the Division of Biological Sciences. Her laboratory combines interests developed during her basic science training in molecular biology and clinical training in reproductive endocrinology and infertility to understand the molecular mechanisms that underlie oocyte and embryo developmental competence in mammals. A major long-term goal of these studies is to improve approaches to diagnose and treat infertility.

Jianping Fu, Ph.D., is an associate professor of mechanical engineering at the University of Michigan, Ann Arbor. His research group integrates micro/nanoengineering, mechanobiology, and stem cell biology for advancing understandings of human development and cancer biology.

Martín García-Castro, Ph.D., is an associate professor of biomedical sciences at the University of California, Riverside. His laboratory focuses on understanding the cellular and molecular mechanisms that govern the formation and differentiation potential of neural crest cells (NCCs). His laboratory aims to uncover and characterize the time, tissues, and molecular pathways regulating NCC formation and to assess the effects of the early environment on NCC differentiation potential. His lab has pioneered work analyzing earlier events in the formation of NCCs in amniotes, and identified Pax7 as a critical transcription factor during early avian neural crest development. They are now investigating its mechanism of action (its regulation, splice variants, interacting partners, and their roles). Dr. García-Castro's lab is using a pan-amniote approach to identify critical mechanisms in early neural crest (NC) development. The lab's research challenges current dogmas and has established new paradigms for studying NC development in diverse species (chick, mouse, rabbit, and human). Its work in birds uses chick and quail embryos to identify the earliest events in NC specification and induction through explant cultures, fate map studies, grafting experiments, expression analysis, and single-cell studies. It is also invested in determining the transcriptional effectors of the signaling pathways it had previously identified as critical for NC induction (BMP, Wnt, and FGF). In mouse embryos the lab is establishing the spatiotemporal expression of early NC markers including critical transcription factors and determining the contribution of Pax7 progenitors to NC derivatives using different transgenic approaches. Dr. García-Castro's lab has adopted the rabbit as an alternative model for mammalian NC development and is investigating basic profiles of expression of NC markers, and for the first time in a mammal his research team is simultaneously investigating NC specification/induction and signaling requirements. To deliver an effective translational approach to human health issues the lab has embraced human NC studies. Importantly, those in Dr. García-Castro's lab have developed a surrogate model of human NC based on human embryonic stem cells, infused by the understanding developed at the lab of early NC biology in model organisms.

Ted Golos, Ph.D., is a professor in and the chair of the Department of Comparative Biosciences in the School of Veterinary Medicine at the University of Wisconsin–Madison. His laboratory works on the biology of the maternal–fetal interface in nonhuman primate models, with particular focus on placental development and function.

Arnold Kriegstein, M.D., Ph.D., is the John Bowes Distinguished Professor in Stem Cell and Tissue Biology and the founding director of the Eli and Edythe Broad Center of Regeneration Medicine and Stem Cell Research at the University of California, San Francisco (UCSF), and a member of the National Academy of Medicine. Dr. Kriegstein received a B.A. from Yale University and his M.D. and Ph.D. from New York University in 1977. He subsequently completed residency training in neurology at the Harvard Brigham and Women's Hospital, Children's Hospital, and Beth Israel Hospital in Boston. He has held academic appointments at Stanford University, Yale University, and Columbia University. In 2004 he joined the Neurology Department at UCSF. Dr. Kriegstein's own research focuses on the way in which neural stem and progenitor cells in the embryonic brain produce neurons and the ways in which this information can be used for cell-based therapies to treat diseases of the nervous system. His lab found that radial glial cells are neuronal stem cells in the developing brain and identified a second type of precursor cell produced by radial glial cells that is responsible for generating specific neuronal subtypes. He has recently begun to characterize the progenitor cells within the developing human brain, where he discovered a novel radial glia subtype that contributes to the huge expansion of neuron number that characterizes human cerebral cortex.

Kathy Niakan, Ph.D., is a group leader at the Francis Crick Institute in London investigating the mechanisms of lineage specification in human embryos and stem cells. Dr. Niakan obtained a B.Sc. in cell and molecular biology and a B.A. in English literature from the University of Washington. She was inspired to pursue molecular biology and genetics following an undergraduate research experience in the laboratory of Wendy Raskind, with the support of a Mary Gates Research Scholarship. She obtained her Ph.D. at University of California, Los Angeles, with Edward McCabe where she researched stem cell and developmental biology and was supported by a National Institutes of Health predoctoral training grant, Paul D. Boyer Fellowship, and a Chancellor's Dissertation Year Fellowship. She was a postdoctoral fellow in the laboratory of Kevin Eggan at Harvard University where she gained experience working with human and mouse pluripotent stem cells and focused on understanding human embryogenesis and the regulation of pluripotency. She then moved to the University of Cambridge as a Centre for Trophoblast Research Next Generation Fellow at the Anne McLaren Laboratory for Regenerative Medicine where she continued to investigate the molecular basis of early cell fate decisions in humans and mice.

Mana Parast, M.D., Ph.D., is a professor in residence in pathology at the University of California, San Diego. She is also a perinatal pathologist and placental biologist. She uses pluripotent stem cells to model and study human trophoblast lineage specification and differentiation in the setting of both normal development and disease.

Martin Pera, Ph.D., is a professor at The Jackson Laboratory in Bar Harbor, Maine. He is an expert in human pluripotent stem cell biology, and his laboratory studies the extrinsic regulation of growth and differentiation of human pluripotent stem cells. The Pera lab uses mouse and human pluripotent stem cells to model neural development, the response of the nervous system to injury, and age-related macular degeneration.

Renee Reijo Pera, Ph.D., is the vice president of research and economic development at the California Polytechnic State University in San Luis Obispo (Cal Poly). Prior to Cal Poly, she served as the vice president for research at Montana State University, was an endowed professor of stem cell biology and regenerative medicine at Stanford University, and a professor at the University of California, San Francisco. Dr. Reijo Pera is an expert on human development, especially the first 6 days of embryonic development and the development of the human germ cell lineage. She has received recognition and awards for her work and teaching from the American Society for Reproductive Medicine, *Time*, *Newsweek*, the Society for the Study of Reproduction, and the National Academy of Inventors.

Nicolas Rivron, Ph.D., is the group leader for the laboratory for synthetic mammalian development at the Institute of Molecular Biotechnology in Vienna. Dr. Rivron is a stem cell biologist and a tissue engineer whose laboratory created the blastoid system, the first model of the pre-implantation conceptus generated solely from stem cells. His laboratory also develops microsystem screening platforms and computational technologies to systematically induce, modulate, and analyze self-organization in vitro.

R. Michael Roberts, D.Phil., is a Chancellor's Professor at the University of Missouri. He is currently an investigator in the Christopher S. Bond Life Sciences Center. He gained his B.A. (1962) and D.Phil. (1965) in plant sciences from Oxford University, England, where he studied root development in corn, but since the mid-1970s has worked primarily as a reproductive biologist. Dr. Roberts is known for his work on uterine secretions, particularly the iron-binding acid phosphatase, uteroferrin, in the pig, and on how the early embryo signals its presence to the mother in ruminant species through the production of small proteins called interferons. He has also studied the role of other unique trophoblast proteins in pregnancy and has (with colleague Jon Green) developed a pregnancy test for cattle which is sold by IDEXX Corp. He made a major transition in research direction in 2003 and began to emphasize the use of pluripotent stem cells to study the emergence and differentiation of trophoblast. His group has also made contributions to the culture of such cells, particularly the importance of low oxygen atmospheres to control differentiation. His was among the first laboratories to describe the generation of induced pluripotent stem cells from an ungulate species, the pig, and it has recently been generating iPS cell lines from human umbilical cords to study preeclampsia. Dr. Roberts was elected to the National Academy of Sciences in 1996 and shared the Wolf Prize in Agriculture in 2003.

Paul Robson, Ph.D., is the director of the Single Cell Biology Laboratory at The Jackson Laboratory in Farmington, Connecticut. He is trained in molecular biology and genetics (B.Sc., University of Guelph), biochemistry (Ph.D., University of Toronto/Sickkids), and developmental biology (postdoc, Children's Hospital of Philadelphia) prior to establishing his developmental cellomics laboratory at the Genome Institute of Singapore

(2002–2014). He joined The Jackson Laboratory for Genomic Medicine in 2014. In Singapore his work focused on elucidating the regulatory networks of early embryonic development and of embryonic stem cells, in mouse and human. In 2010 his interests in gaining a molecular understanding of cell fate decisions led to one of the first studies employing single-cell gene expression technologies. Since then he has continued to apply such technologies to understand the biology of early development, cancer, and immunology. Current research interests include using human pluripotent cells to model and study human peri-implantation biology with a focus on human/simian-specific features.

Janet Rossant, Ph.D., FRS, FRSC, is the president and the scientific director of the Gairdner Foundation and a senior scientist and the chief of research emeritus at The Hospital for Sick Children in Toronto. She is an internationally recognized developmental and stem cell biologist who explores the origins of stem cells in the early embryo and their applications to understanding and treating human disease.

Aryeh Warmflash, Ph.D., is an assistant professor of bioscеiences and bioengineering at Rice University. He received his Ph.D. in physics at the University of Chicago and did postdoctoral training at The Rockefeller University. His lab uses human embryonic stem cells to study early embryonic development quantitatively.

Jun Wu, Ph.D., is an assistant professor in the Department of Molecular Biology at the University of Texas Southwestern Medical Center, Dallas. Dr. Wu's work has contributed to the generation of new stem cells for basic and translational studies and to developing novel and efficient genome and epigenome editing tools. His group is particularly interested in harnessing stem cell–derived interspecies chimeras and synthetic embryos for studying early mammalian development, pluripotency and molecular mechanisms of xenogeneic barriers.

Magdalena Zernicka-Goetz, Ph.D., is a professor of mammalian development and stem cell biology at the University of Cambridge and the Bren Professor of Biology and Biological Engineering at the California Institute of Technology. Dr. Zernicka-Goetz carried out her Ph.D. at the University of Warsaw, Poland, under supervision of Andrzej Tarkowski. She moved to Cambridge in 1995 to join the Martin Evans group with the long-term aim of studying the mechanisms of regulative nature of development and spatial patterning in the mouse embryo. In 1997 she was awarded a Senior Research Fellowship from the Lister Institute to start her independent group at the Wellcome Trust/Cancer Research UK Gurdon Institute in Cambridge. In 2001 she became a Wellcome Senior Research Fellow. In 2010 she became a professor of mammalian development and stem cell biology. She received a Promising Young Scientist Prize from Foundation for Polish Science in 1993 and a Young Investigator Award from the European Molecular Biology Organization (EMBO) in 2001, was elected to EMBO membership in 2007, and became a fellow of the British Academy of Medical Science in 2013.

Appendix C

Statement of Task

A planning committee of the National Academies of Sciences, Engineering, and Medicine will organize and conduct a 1-day public workshop to explore the state of the science of mammalian embryo model systems, including nonhuman primate and human models. The goal of the workshop will be to begin with an overview of the developments and uses that have set the foundation for the field, then to focus in on opportunities and challenges for future work with embryo model systems. Discussions may include topics such as the characteristics of advanced mammalian embryo model systems; differences between various mammalian embryo model systems and bona fide mammalian embryos; and differences between mammalian embryo model systems and mammalian "embryoid bodies" (culture systems in which pluripotent stem cells aggregate and differentiate, but the cells are not organized in the same manner as in a bona fide embryo). Discussion may include whether the embryo model systems, especially those using nonhuman primate cells, could be used to predict function of systems made with human cells. The functionality and organismal potential of the synthetic models may be considered, including whether embryo model systems have organismal potential if they lack trophoblast cells or other extraembryonic cell types. The current state of the science of the in vitro development of human trophoblast cells may be considered. As requested by the National Institutes of Health, the discussions at the workshop will focus on the state of the science and not policy or ethical implications given the existing legal limitations. Presentations during this workshop will be held with a broad array of invited stakeholders which may include research scientists from government, academia and the private sector, societies and associations, and representatives from pharmaceutical and biotech companies. The planning committee will develop the workshop agenda, select and invite speakers, and moderate the discussions. Proceedings from the workshop will be prepared by a designated rapporteur in accordance with institutional policies and procedures.

Appendix D

Registered Attendees

Diaa Ahmed
Utrecht University

Eric Anthony
International Society for Stem Cell Research

Jeannie Baumann
Bloomberg Law

Lizbet Boroughs
Association of American Universities

Amir Brivanlou
Kenyon College

Nima Brivanlou
University of St. Andrews

Liza Bundesen
National Institutes of Health

Carlo Carvalho
SIMR

Naomi Charalambakis
Federation of American Societies for Experimental Biology

Clara Cheng
National Institutes of Health/ National Institute of Child Health and Human Development

Irene Cheng
National Institutes of Health

Ida Chow
Society for Developmental Biology

Justin Cotney
University of Connecticut

James Coulombe
National Institutes of Health/
National Institute of
Child Health and Human
Development

Catherine Domingo
National Cancer Institute

Jennifer Dumdie
University of California, San Diego

Tuba Fehr
National Institutes of Health/
National Institute of
Child Health and Human
Development

Ellen Gadbois
National Institutes of Health

Kenneth Gibbs
National Institutes of Health/
National Institute of General
Medical Sciences

Norbert Gleicher
Center for Human Reproduction

Andrew Guernsey
U.S. Senator Steve Daines

Dianne Hardy
National Institutes of Health/
Center for Scientific Review

Deborah Henken
National Institutes of Health

Tanya Hoodbhoy
National Institutes of Health

Gary Hunnicutt
National Institutes of Health

Anna Jacobs
National Institutes of Health

Lyric Jorgenson
National Institutes of Health

Lisa Kaeser
National Institutes of Health/
National Institute of
Child Health and Human
Development

Kym Kilbourne
International Society for Stem
Cell Research

Louise Laurent
University of California, San Diego

Zukai Liu
The Jackson Laboratory

Lynn Marquis
Coalition for the Life Sciences

Joseph McKenna
National Institutes of Health/
National Cancer Institute

Stephanie Miceli
National Academies of Sciences,
Engineering, and Medicine/
Office of News and Public
Information

Jack Mosher
International Society for Stem Cell
Research

Stuart Moss
National Institutes of Health/
National Institute of
Child Health and Human
Development

Mahua Mukhopadhyay
National Institutes of Health

Teresa Olbrich
National Institutes of Health/
National Cancer Institute

John O'Shea
National Institutes of Health/
National Institute of Arthritis
and Musculoskeletal and Skin
Diseases

David Owens
National Institutes of Health/
National Institute of
Neurological Disorders and
Stroke

Erica Pandolfi
University of California, Los
Angeles

Chanel Press
National Institutes of Health

Beverly Purnell
American Association for the
Advancement of Science/
Science magazine

Heather Randall
Independent

Neelakanta Ravindranath
National Institutes of Health/
National Institute of
Child Health and Human
Development

Antonio Regalado
MIT Technology Review

Pamela Robey
National Institutes of Health/
National Institute of Dental
and Craniofacial Research

Sergio Macias Ruiz
National Institutes of Health

Pierre Savatier
INSERM

Kelly Servick
Science magazine

Elaine Sierra-Rivera
National Institutes of Health

Aparna Singh
National Institutes of Health

Lilianna Solnica-Krezel
Washington University School
of Medicine in St. Louis

Kathryn Stein
National Institutes of Health/
National Institute of Dental
and Craniofacial Research

Nidhi Subbaraman
Nature

Yuliana Tan
The Jackson Laboratory for Genomic Medicine

Susan Taymans
National Institutes of Health/National Institute of Child Health and Human Development

Thorold Theunissen
Washington University School of Medicine in St. Louis

Reiko Toyama
National Institutes of Health/National Institute of Child Health and Human Development

Jessica Tucker
National Institutes of Health/Office of Science Policy

Maria Sendino Vega
National Institutes of Health

Sissy Wamaitha
University of California, Los Angeles

Ellen Wann
National Institutes of Health

Kelvin Wilson
American Society for Cell Biology

Carrie Wolinetz
National Institutes of Health